Cancer's Cause, Cancer's Cure

The Truth About Cancer, Its Causes, Cures, and Prevention

Morton Walker, D.P.M.

Hugo House Publishers, Ltd.

Cancer's Cause, Cancer's Cure: The Truth about Cancer, its Causes, Cures, and Prevention

ISBN: 978-1-936449-10-1

Library of Congress Control Number: 2012933207

Cover Design/Interior Layout: NZ Graphics

PCIP listing: pending

Hugo House Publishers, Ltd.
Englewood, Colorado
Austin, Texas
(877) 700-0616
www.HugoHousePublishers.com

First Edition

Printed in the United States of America

To Joan Bloom Walker, my beloved wife.

At age sixty-eight, Joan succumbed to inflammatory breast disease, the deadly carcinoma showing a five-year patient survival rate of just 1.5 percent. In spite of an exhaustive search and trial worldwide for natural and non-toxic therapies (fifty-two of them), the patient and her loved ones failed to reverse the cancer that eventually killed Joan on February 4, 2000.

We did not know of Dr. Mirko Beljanski's discoveries when Joan was afflicted; however, I sincerely believe that making use of the new information presented in this text definitely would have contributed to saving her life.

Acknowledgments

To Sylvie Beljanski and Monique Beljanski, the daughter and the wife of Mirko Beljanski, Ph.D., as well as the entire CIRIS team. These two women introduced me to the *Centre d'Innovations, de Recherches et d'Informations Scientifiques* (CIRIS), a French healthcare membership organization, and then offered numerous recorded interviews about the professional life and works of their incredibly creative kin, Dr. Beljanski, the deceased scientific genius discussed here.

To Michael Baybak, whom I consulted as my literary agent but who swiftly became a truly valued friend. Michael exhibited faith in eight-and-a-half years of investigations I had conducted on Dr. Mirko Beljanski and turned my written conclusions into a published book.

To my son Randall Scott Walker, who supported me with supplementary research on the Beljanski concept of cancer's causation and its cure.

To holistic physician Michael B. Schachter, MD, who introduced me to Dr. Beljanski's daughter and wife and then contributed innumerable hours—even days, to editing this book for medical and scientific accuracy.

To George Gluchowski, President and copublisher of Hugo House Publishers, Ltd. who envisions this book's information as a primary source of prolonged human health by the elimination of cancer and other degenerative diseases in our lifetime.

To copublisher Patricia Ross, Ph.D., who rearranged editorial content. Even with my having produced over ninety published books, I learned much from the editorship of Dr. Ross. It was my joy to work with Patricia, and I hope to do so again.

To my significant other (SO) Sheila M. Bruck, who assisted me with copyediting this work.

Table of Contents

Disclaimer

The purpose of this book is to educate. The author and/or publisher do not guarantee that anyone following these techniques, suggestions, tips, ideas, or strategies will engender success. The author and/or publisher shall have neither liability nor responsibility to anyone with respect to any loss or damage caused, or alleged to be caused, directly or indirectly by the information contained in this book.

The information in this book is not medical advice. Seek the advice of a qualified and caring physician, naturopath, homeopath, or other certified medical specialist before embarking on any health-care regime.

This book has been written and published strictly for informational purposes, and in no way should be used as a substitute for advice from your own health-care professional.

You must not consider educational material found here as a replacement for consultation with medical, osteopathic, homeopathic, dental, naturopathic, chiropractic, podiatric, acupuncture, nutritional, nursing, or other types of health-care practitioners.

The facts in our text come from laboratory and/or clinical studies, scientific publications, interviews with informed health-care personnel, and interviews of patients who have experienced the herbal and dietary supplements described herein.

Unless otherwise indicated, as by footnotes or parenthetical insertions, the identities of patients cited here are true and not pseudonyms, including the individuals' occupations, residences or locations, plus their direct quotes. The patients' descriptions of signs and symptoms of illnesses are true and may be accessed for verification by contacting those health professionals who discuss their patients. Direct quotes of health-care practitioners are taken from tape recorded interviews or from published research papers, text books, consumer books, and/or contributed press clippings for our inclusion.

If information gleaned here raises questions about your own, a loved one's, or an acquaintance's health and wellness, please consult your own knowledgeable medical expert. The author works as a medical journalist and is *not* an expert on medical, dental, chiropractic, osteopathic, or other health care. To be clear in our advisory, the author states that he is a freelance medical journalist who depends on health-professional authorities or other medical-type experts and their patients for information. The author gains knowledge by use of literature on the subject, one-on-one personal interviews, in-person medical/dental reportorial investigations, and the incorporation of such investigations into his finished writings.

Please take the above message as a disavowal of all responsibility by the author, consultants, publisher, editorial content contributors, cited organizations, and product suppliers for any medical device, practice, procedure, dietary program, nutritional supplement, diagnostic technique, or other information taken from this publication and acted upon by readers or other interested parties.

Preface

Cancer. A disease that has stalked us, haunted us, killed our loved ones, and made us cry for mercy as we've emptied our pocketbooks to fight it. In the 1960s, the Nixon administration declared war on this most feared disease. I have long thought that perhaps this is the one war we can't win even as we continue to fight against the increasingly insurmountable odds of a cure.

Collectively, we're tired, bone tired. We have had our hopes continually hyped and then dashed by the promise of cure after cure. The medical establishment has been both sanctified and vilified because of the hundreds of thousands of research hours and multi billions of dollars spent trying to understand and fight this scourge effectively. Trillions have been wasted on failed medicines. Alternative medicine, for which I am a proponent and outspoken representative, has offered its own treatments, some effective; many abysmal failures.

Has all this time and money done anything? That's hard to say. Sometimes I wonder who's at war with whom. Are we all fighting for the same cause—to finally find a way to best conquer this most dreaded of killers? Or are we fighting each other—the medical establishment clashing against alternative holistic practitioners? A villainous faction of the medical establishment has long been accused of making cancer into big business. This faction has sided with the large pharmaceutical companies and their powerful lobbies, who oftentimes and with derision are called, "Big Pharma," and together they have had the charge leveled against them that they ultimately do not want to find a cure because that would cut off the billions in funding they both receive.

Those caught in the middle of this massive and expensive assault—the everyday person who either has to fight cancer or who has to watch a loved one succumb—witness all the posturing and politicizing and wonder why. Why must this madness continue when there's something so precious that we're losing, day after day, year in and year out—our lives?

Nearly ten years ago, I retired from my active participation in medical journalism. But when cancer took my wife, my mother, my sister, and my fiancée who had pledged to spend her last years with me, I knew I had to step up and not only uncover which alternatives really worked but let the world know about it.

It has taken me almost a decade to find and articulate the answer, an answer that had been in existence for many years prior to my beloved wife's death, an answer that has been thoroughly researched and tested, not by a doctor or a big pharmaceutical research-and-development team, but by a humble scientist who had found himself caught in the cross hairs of French politics and science, a man who had worked for twenty-five years at the famed Pasteur Institute in Paris as a microbiologist, a hero genius who was relentless in discovering how cancer works at the very foundation of life, the DNA of our cells.

In short, this book presents concepts, discoveries, and specific approaches to correct deadly illnesses, in particular cancer, developed from the research studies of French biochemist and molecular biologist, Mirko Beljanski, Ph.D. But that dry description belies the enormous gesture of help that this one man has offered humanity.

Dr. Beljanski, deceased since October 1998, was a Yugoslavian-born French citizen. When he was forced to leave the Pasteur Institute, he didn't stop working. He pursued two more decades of independent research on the restoration of human homeostasis (the body's natural push for internal stability). He didn't want to see people die, and he knew he could do something about it.

Throughout his life, he made significant and vital breakthroughs in his search for the causes of degenerative disease and was on the verge of other equally significant findings at his death. Most important, our hero's quest for knowledge led him to significant discoveries in the fields of cancer and viral illnesses including the reversal of signs and symptoms of cancer, AIDS, hepatitis C, and herpes. His intent was to sustain people at their normal condition of good health. His findings deserve the highest accolades anyone can give another human being.

Beljanski used fundamental science to investigate gene activation and inactivation, all manner of cell division and tissue development in both normal and abnormal states, plus the basic fundamentals of life. In accordance with Dr. Beljanski's beliefs, he searched for ways to restore good health in the general population through cellular balance, and his research tended towards the use of available natural substances instead of turning to synthetic compounds such as prescribed medications, over-the-counter drugs, or any other type of chemicalized synthetic therapies.

As the ultimate man of science, he was holistic in his orientation and believed in alternative forms of healing from natural and non-toxic sources. He represented the scientific method in its truest form.

Work began for him at the Pasteur Institute with his pioneering studies in RNA (ribonucleic acid), one of the basic building blocks of a cell and thus of all life. Over his professional career of more than forty-five years, Dr. Beljanski brought to light the negative impact environmental pollution has on human, animal, and plant health at the DNA level. He discovered what happens to a cell at the molecular level, thereby discovering the DNA of cancer. Once he understood how a cell becomes cancerous, he was able to find and perfect the application of anticancer and antiviral botanical approaches which, if used properly, can handle most cancers.

Yes, you read that correctly—I believe these botanical approaches can cure most cancers. I do not say that lightly because I know of what I speak. As a medical journalist, I have dedicated my life to bringing to the public important discoveries in holistic medicine. I have published ninety-one other books on consumer health, and I believe this book you're reading, number ninety-two, is my most momentous. I came out of retirement because I know that what Dr. Mirko Beljanski discovered could save millions of lives. His discoveries could put an end to the war on cancer.

My Introduction to Dr. Beljanski's Concepts

Dr. Beljanski's discoveries need to be brought to broad public attention so that we all can be better informed if we or someone we love develops cancer or contracts an incurable virus. If we understand how cancer develops in our bodies, we can better understand why Beljanski's break-through discoveries are so effective.

My introduction to Mirko Beljanski happened in the spring of 2003, when I attended the semi-annual scientific conference of the American College for Advancement in Medicine (ACAM), an organization of twenty-five hundred holistic medical practitioners. There I listened to a lecture by Michael B. Schachter, M.D., of Suffern, New York. Trained in a form of holistic psychiatry which uses nutrients rather than drugs for treating mental illness, Dr. Schachter works as a holistic physician with alternative methods of healing and has administered to thousands of patients for close to forty years. He is renowned among his colleagues, loved by his patients, and has vast experience with therapies that do no harm when overcoming serious infirmities. Most of his patients consult him, not for mind-related disturbances, but for cancer, cardiovascular, and peripheral vascular diseases (blood clots), in addition to other serious health issues. His patients usually need no hospitalization and no drug prescriptions. Typically they take nutritional supplements in addition to following wholesome diets.

I knew Dr. Schachter from when my wife, Joan, came down with breast cancer and suffered its subsequent required mastectomy in 1987; Dr. Schachter kept her healthy, beautiful, and thriving for over thirteen years. Joan taught nutrition, diet, weight control, and positive thinking to thousands of women throughout Connecticut. She was their mentor, and I was never more proud of my beautiful wife.

It was not ordinary breast cancer that killed my wife eventually but rather something much worse—inflammatory breast disease. Because I was unaware of Dr. Beljanski's products, I like everyone else believed that no treatment of any kind had ever been found for her illness. The condition killed her within ten months of its diagnosis.

Cancer is an indiscriminate grim reaper, and I was destined to suffer more loss at its menacing hands. Three months after Joan's funeral, my mother, Rachel Walker, was diagnosed with gastric carcinoma (cancer of the stomach). Having no knowledge that she was afflicted, I had left the country. With a heavy heart, I was required to fly home at once to arrange for her burial.

After living the lonely life of a widower for three years, I received a call. It was Dr. Schachter, inviting me to come to the 2003 ACAM conference. My respect for Dr. Schachter has been immense for as long as I've known him—at least twenty-seven years—and I knew that any medical topic he would present in a lecture was worthwhile to hear. So when he invited me to listen to his talk on the cancer-causation concepts of Dr. Mirko Beljanski, I sensed in advance that my time spent at the ACAM conference would be significant.

The holistic physician introduced me to Monique and Sylvie Beljanski, the wife and the daughter of Dr. Beljanski. They had also listened to Dr. Schachter's presentation. In turn, the two women invited me to a beautiful part of France called Charente to attend a picnic, scheduled for September 5, 2003, conducted by the "Center of Innovation, Research and Scientific Information" (*Centre d'Innovation, de Recherches et d'Information Scientifiques*: CIRIS). CIRIS is an organization with a membership between thirty-five hundred and five thousand French men and women, all of whom had been saved from cancer or AIDS by application of Dr. Beljanski's discoveries and the concept of cancer causation surrounding them.

By April 2003, Dr. Schachter had informed CIRIS and the Beljanski women that my publishing score was eighty-six distributed consumer health books to my credit. Their idea was that I might become intrigued with the knowledge I acquired in La Rochelle, France, and write a book on the professional life and work of Dr. Mirko Beljanski. I was astounded by what I found and believed I had come across knowledge about the most viable weapons to date to fight cancer.

Shortly after I returned from the picnic in France where I learned of Beljanski's work, I discovered my sister, Phyllis Greene, had lung cancer. She suffered terrible discomforts arising from undergoing the usual oncological (the branch of medicine dealing with cancer) treatments of radiation and chemotherapy. Radiation therapy causes burns to the skin and/or brings on diarrhea of the gastrointestinal tract. Chemotherapy commonly produces nausea, vomiting, loss of appetite, weight loss, depression, fatigue, low red-blood cell counts that lead to anemia and low white blood-cell counts that promote the risk of infection. From receiving chemotherapy, people often lose their hair or experience inflammation or ulcers of the mucous membranes, such as the mouth lining, which makes eating difficult. Phyllis experienced all of these until she longed for death, whereupon she entered a hospice in anticipation of the end.

I brought Beljanski's products for my sister to ingest. She took them gratefully and benefited from them. The various formulas derived from nature reduced my sister's awful chemotherapeutic side effects. I visited her weekly, even though the round trip to see her was an eight-hour drive. Her oncologist took credit for his patient's improvement, and neither my sister nor I corrected his taking such credit.

When the local chapter of Hospice in Sebring, Florida, learned that Phyllis' improvement came from the herbals I was leaving, her hospice nurses and aides took them away. I was outraged and discovered that the Institution of Hospice requires that nothing be done for the dying patient to allow his or her lingering in this life on earth. Everything is done to ease the patient into the next life. Even the removal of cancer treatment that gives comfort seems to be mandatory.

My sister quickly succumbed to the lung cancer. I believe that she would be with us still if she had continued to take Beljanski's botanicals. I vowed at her death that I would make sure the world knew about this amazing man and the potential his anti-cancer botanicals, developed through meticulous microbiological research, held for humanity. I never wanted to see another loved one suffer. But that was not to be.

Before my sister died, I met a kind and attractive woman, and having been a widower for three years, I opened myself to love again. We dated for several months, and then we took a tour together to nine cities in Spain. I traveled there with an engagement ring in my pocket.

We planned to be married within the early months of 2005. Instead, during the late fall and early winter of 2004, I frequented the reception areas and consultation rooms of Massachusetts General Hospital (MGH), a major teaching institution in Boston, because my fiancée had been admitted to this hospital with pancreatic cancer. Such cancer is an illness with a devastating prognosis, for it has no screening technique; therefore less than 7 percent of cases are detected early. The rest are spotted when pain or other symptoms appear. Some 37,680 new cases of pancreatic cancer occurred in 2008, with a mere 2 percent experiencing a five-year survival rate. [1]

During meetings with some oncologists and radiotherapists who were responsible for the care of this woman to whom I had newly proposed marriage, I was astounded at how distorted the physicians' presentations were when they discussed the side effects of their treatments. The doctors appeared to become almost like used-car salesmen in a pitch for their surgery, radiation therapy and/or chemotherapy. I know something about medical practices and oncology from my work as a medical researcher and as a former practicing podiatrist. In my opinion, the information the oncologists gave my fiancée was hardly an honest assessment of the relative benefits and risks associated with the recommended treatments.

My fiancée, her two educated, middle-age sons, and I consulted twice with a group of oncological specialists employed by the hospital. The decision was made that this sixty-six-year-old woman, diagnosed with an aggressive pancreatic cancer, required immediate surgery employing the Whipple's operation triad. The Whipple's is a very extensive operative procedure that involves the excision of at least three internal organs, including a majority of the victim's pancreas.

To prepare the woman's internal cancerous tissues, preoperative radiation was recommended for her, and following operative recovery, postoperative chemotherapy was also mandatory. Both radiation and chemotherapy oncologists went about selling their separate treatments to the patient, her sons, and me. When I asked about the residual side effects of the typical treatment, her oncologists told us that there were none. My fiancée, her sons, and I were astounded. "No side effects? How could that be?" The oncologists were steadfast in their declarations. I knew they were lying.

When my fiancée and I arrived for her required preoperative radiation, I observed literally hundreds of bald-headed women waiting in the radiotherapy and chemotherapy hospital areas for commencement of their next treatments. I thought, with no small amount of disgust, "Isn't the loss of hair with resultant baldheadedness a side effect of one or both of these cancer therapies?" All of us know that it is. I was also dismayed as I watched these unfortunate people running into the conveniently placed toilets—one toilet bowl for approximately every twelve reception room chairs—to vomit.

I was opposed to the radiation therapy, but that's what this patient and her two sons elected for her to do. I tried to convince her to check into a program run by a friend, a holistic oncologist named Nicholas J. Gonzalez, M.D., of New York City. Dr. Gonzalez was ready to take her into the program. The Gonzalez patient investigations had been funded by the U.S. Government as a successful clinical-research program that uses certain types of enzymes derived from New Zealand lambs. She refused Dr. Gonzalez's offer. (Please see Appendix A for more information about Dr. Gonzalez's pancreatic cancer-reversal program.)

I also had Beljanski's supplements. I was not forceful in pressing for use of those holistic products. I cooperated with the others' treatment decision. When I finally encouraged my fiancée to take Dr. Beljanski's botanicals, I was hopeful, but they were soon abandoned. Her two sons, a stock broker and a computer programmer, would have none of my recommendations. My fiancée and her sons did not understand how and why they worked. Beljanski's herbals ended up being flushed down the hospital room's toilet. They considered holistic-type therapies outright quackery.

Condemned by these young men, I was literally ordered to leave the hospital scene. In fact, they insisted I leave Massachusetts altogether. They said, "Get out of our mother's life! Go home to Connecticut!" She died within two months of her sons sending me away.

Granted, the track record for pancreatic cancer is poor for virtually all known treatments, whether conventional or alternative. However, I personally have met scores of former cancer patients taking Beljanski's very safe supplements who had been given short-term death sentences by their doctors years prior, including pancreatic cancer. So it is my belief that if my former fiancée had accepted and tried Dr. Beljanski's natural and non-toxic discoveries, she might still be with us today.

I am certain that most of you who are reading this book have lost someone you loved—a family member, a friend, a beloved teacher or mentor—to cancer. Don't we all deserve to know about a way to treat cancer effectively, without pain, and for extended periods of time?

An Integrative Approach

The traditional treatment for cancer is well-known. Radiation therapy and chemotherapy are designed to kill the cancerous cells. The problem is that the treatment oftentimes kills the patient. Radiation and harsh chemicals do not discriminate between good and bad cells—the treatments kill all cells. Three renown oncologists reporting in the peer-reviewed medical journal *Clinical Oncology* declared that "the benefit of cytotoxic (a substance having a fatal effect on cells) chemotherapy may have been overestimated for cancers of the esophagus, stomach, rectum, and brain with a minimal impact of cytotoxic chemotherapy on five-year survival, and a lack of any major progress over the last twenty years." In other words, doctors who are trained to treat cancer are saying that the conventional treatments they use are not working—at least not as well as some would like everyone to believe.

When I started my research on Mirko Beljanski, Ph.D., I was determined that I would use his findings as a way to warn my readers away from conventionally administered cancer therapies. Radiation treatment assuredly burns any tissues it touches, and chemicals given as cancer therapy produce adverse side effects of one's metabolism so awful, they often cause the patient eventually to wish for death. I have long advocated for my readers to avoid them because nearly all of their applications are deadly, damaging, and costly; plus they deteriorate the quality of life for someone who is already at death's door.

I am a doctor of podiatric medicine (D.P.M.), but as a full-time medical journalist for the past forty-plus years, my advice is, and has always been, to seek the services of a holistic-oriented health-care professional such as a naturopath, a homeopath, an acupuncturist, or an herbalist who keeps you out of the hospital or who uses very few pharmaceutical products or no drugs at all.

I have especially been outspoken against the pharmaceutical industry, the companies who make the drugs as well as their powerful lobbyists. I stand firm with Dr. Julian Whitaker, who in his March 2011 *Health & Healing*® monthly newsletter, wrote: "The pharmaceutical industry makes the most dangerous products on the planet. Prescription meds are our fourth leading cause of death, and some of them have unthinkable side effects. Psychiatric drugs, for instance, have been linked to countless suicides, school shootings, and other bizarre acts of violence such as mothers killing their own children.

"The large drug companies are cash cows. According to Fortune 500 rankings, their mean profit margin is 20 percent, compared to an 8 percent average across all industries... Big Pharma gets irrational sweetheart deals from the government. For Medicare prescription drug coverage, prices are not negotiable. They [Big Pharma] can charge the government whatever they want!

"This industry spends nearly twice as much on advertising as they do on research and development. Direct-to-consumer advertising, which is allowed only in the U.S. and New Zealand, has created unprecedented demand for medications, driven up usage and profits, and corrupted the doctor-patient relationship." [3]

You can verify Dr. Julian Whitaker's statements by just turning on your television set. Over half of the ads on television it seems are for one kind of drug or another. It makes you wonder why the drug companies need to promote their drugs so heavily.

While cancer drugs are not advertised, it is an irrefutable fact that chemotherapy and radiation currently being prescribed by oncologists world-wide are unable to effectively distinguish between cells to be destroyed and cells to be preserved. For this reason at the present time, a "cure" for cancer does not exist and frequently the establishment's treatment is as deadly as the disease.

But this is what makes Dr. Beljanski's approach so important. You can imagine my surprise when I learned that Dr. Beljanski's supplements, while amazingly effective on their own, when coupled with *low* doses of radiation and chemotherapy, are effective, *perhaps more so than any other combined treatment available.*

I was astounded.

I am holistic to the core of my being, but Beljanski was a meticulous researcher, constantly probing the depths of what was known and unknown about cancer at the cellular level. His discoveries work because they are selective against a collection of cellular deviations identified as a *malignancy,* a *mass,* a *tumor,* a *growth,* or a *cancer.* In the course of destroying the illness, Beljanski's botanicals target the cancerous cells. Not only do they suppress or destroy cancer cells, but they also distinguish harmful cells from healthy ones and thereby leave healthy cells undamaged. His approach is different from anything offered by modern oncology.

Mirko Beljanski's research took him to the very core of our physical life—to the basic building blocks of DNA and its close kin, RNA. He discovered what happens to the DNA of a cancer cell and how that can be rectified to bring about that all important balance in the human cell. His research into RNA was revolutionary at a time when RNA was relegated to the back burners of most laboratories, including the Pasteur; it yielded results that in our modern day of incurable diseases are indispensable.

This is a highly important subject—vital for the saving of lives—and I consider myself privileged to bring it to you. Beljanski's anticancer approach is scientifically based, tested, and proven both in the laboratory and in human clinical trials. If indeed we are at war against cancer and not against each other, if we are truly going to best this scourge that according to most accounts is worsening across the globe, then it is time to put aside our differences, look at the evidence at hand, and soldier ahead. For we *can* win this war on cancer if we let the discoveries of Dr. Mirko Beljanski lead the way.

Introduction

In the spring of 1992, Jean-Paul Le Perlier, a French journalist known for his forthright news editorials in political journals and newspapers along with five national bestselling books, was contacted by his closest friend. This friend also just happened to be a major figure in the world of the international pharmaceutical companies. The drug-company executive asked Monsieur Le Perlier if he would investigate one Dr. Mirko Beljanski. Why? Because his drug company's sales were being adversely affected by certain products Beljanski created. This friend claimed the microbiologist was a "quack" and wanted Le Perlier to write an exposé on Beljanski and publish it in the widely circulated political journal that Le Perlier worked for, *Minute.*

I met Monsieur Le Perlier at the CIRIS picnic I was invited to attend by Sylvie and Monique Beljanski (CIRIS stands for the *Center of Scientific Innovations, Research, and Information*).[4] They had asked me to come to France earlier that year in 2003 at the ACAM (American College of Advancement in Medicine) convention where I had learned about Dr. Beljanski's work.[5] The picnic, held in La Rochelle, France, on September 5, 2003, was attended by several hundred people, but I was there to interview prior cancer victims who had used Beljanski's products and who no longer suffered from cancer. I wanted to find out for myself how effective they really were.

At the time of my arrival in La Rochelle there were 3,522 officially recorded members of CIRIS plus another approximately two thousand formerly ill people who frequently attended meetings but did not pay dues. Almost all of these official and non-official attendees should have been dead from oncological or other degenerative illnesses one, two, or three decades before. Instead, many hundreds of them were present at the CIRIS picnic, and all in all, I interviewed three dozen former cancer patients. Each gave me written permission to use what they revealed about themselves.

The CIRIS members had paid my travel expenses and met me with smiling faces and open arms. The members' goal was to convince me that the message they wanted delivered in book form had the potential to save millions of people from a variety of serious degenerative diseases.

I had been told that Le Perlier's story was especially important because he had information about President François Mitterrand, France's president from 1981 through 1995, who had allegedly taken Beljanski's formulas for his prostate cancer.

I wondered what had happened to Le Perlier that transformed him from a highly conservative medical skeptic to a true believer of holistic methods of health care. Cheating death is a powerful motivator for change, however, and that is exactly what happened to Le Perlier. It turns out, he saved his own life by using Dr. Beljanski's products. I needed to know the full story.

The Personal Story of Journalist Jean-Paul Le Perlier

It is often said that truth is stranger than fiction, and that is most definitely the case with Jean-Paul Le Perlier. His story is so utterly fantastic that I must relate his narrative to you, transcribed from a tape recorder, most of it word for word:

"My best friend, who has rendered me enormous service and for whom I can refuse nothing, just happened to be the executive vice president of the French subsidiary of a major international manufacturer of chemotherapeutic agents," began the famous French journalist. "My friend represents the interests of pharmaceuticals throughout Europe and the United States of America, including the Pharmaceutical Research and Manufacturers of America (the powerful lobby otherwise known to some as Big Pharma).

"During our visit together in the spring of 1992," Le Perlier continued, "my friend advised that his drug company's product sales were being adversely affected by a particular molecular biologist he referred to as 'fraudulent and a quack.' Knowing that I am a journalist, my friend asked me to do him a favor and undertake a journalistic investigation—write a special exposé on this 'scoundrel' whom he identified as 'Mirko Beljanski, Ph.D.'

"And," Le Perlier added with emphasis, "this vice president for the international drug company's subsidiary told me, 'It's thought by some people that Beljanski's products are curing cancer. Of course, this cannot be true because for decades pharmaceutical companies have attempted to do the same thing, but they have obviously failed. There is no cure, but numbers of medical consumers think this Beljanski faker has produced some kind of treatment to correct not only cancer but also AIDS. Certainly that thinking is nonsense when everyone knows that drugs, cytotoxic agents (substances that are toxic to cells), and other chemotherapies manufactured by my industry remain unsuccessful. If the pharmaceutical companies cannot cure cancer, then no one and nothing can do it.'"

Le Perlier made it clear that his friend was adamant: "'Moreover, the simultaneous treatment of cancer and AIDS is obvious quackery,' continued my friend, 'since any knowledgeable person recognizes that a single set of products can't be used for two dissimilar illnesses. With cancer coming from the body's interior and AIDS contracted from its exterior, it's absolutely impossible to conceive that one therapy would be useful for both. Beljanski must be a charlatan because with this scoundrel lecturing publicly, his is a ridicule of France's scientific works. We in French drug manufacturing cannot put up with that snake-oil salesman's offensive nostrum-peddling.'

"Consequently," Le Perlier continued, speaking for himself now, "the drug company executive called upon me to warn people away from giving credence to research coming from this maverick professor. It was not difficult for me to see the advantages of producing an exposé article or even a series of articles. I figured it to be an easy assignment to accomplish.

"Since I am a journalist, and it was my responsibility to fill a full newspaper page of copy in the broadly-circulated French weekly political gazette, *Minute*, I could offer space for an exposé of Dr. Beljanski along with his so-called cancer- and AIDS-curing botanicals. Whether in politics or in health, I see my job as defending the interests of consumers," Le Perlier stated firmly. "Incidentally, *Minute* with its political issues has now on September 7, 2003, gone out of print and is no longer published. When I brought this article assignment to my editors, however, they agreed that I should quickly move on the story.

"The editors' joint decision was to have me *not* directly interview Beljanski; rather, my work must be dedicated to interviewing patients and to writing the story of only a few cancer victims who were using his treatments," Le Perlier advised. "The editors' intent was to have me speak to at least twenty-five of the patients and select two or three whose health I judged were being severely hurt by Beljanski. I expected to keep in touch with these unfortunates all the way through to their deaths, so that in follow-up articles my newspaper would be free from any possible lawsuits that evolved from publication of our ongoing exposé.

"My deadline to produce the first article was in two weeks. Consequently, I quickly sought out doctors and nurses who could put me in contact with cancer patients using Beljanski's supplements," continued Le Perlier. "I wanted to speak with any person who had negative statements to offer about them; only, I couldn't find any. After fourteen days of interviewing, there were no contrary reports; the product users were happy and thriving. I failed to meet my deadline, and it became necessary for me to pull a previously written piece out of inventory and run that less-relevant article at the end of two weeks. Although I wanted badly to blast Beljanski, I had nothing to write that would condemn his practices or his products.

"I interviewed more Beljanski product-users for another two weeks, and the lack of disgruntled customers left me thwarted and feeling frustrated. Still, because of the promise I had made to my drug industry friend, the Beljanski investigation for me went on for several months more. Not one person during the entire time had anything negative to say about Dr. Beljanski's discoveries. My published articles continued to contain nothing about that annoying molecular biologist," Le Perlier said, smirking at the memory.

"Even so, my *Minute* page of copy had to be filled, and enthusiasm for the story died among my editors. Upon the newspaper's managing editor expressing disappointment with the absence of any Beljanski exposé, I renewed my search for that scientist's skullduggery by devoting about fifteen non-productive hours each week to the investigation for the balance of 1992," Le Perlier told me.

Drugstore Owners Sue Beljanski

"Early the next year news came to me that a lawsuit brought by pharmacists on behalf of the Republic of France was ongoing against Dr. Beljanski in the southern city of Saint-Etienne. Plaintiffs' attorneys claimed that the molecular biologist was using drugs illegally, and the sales of legitimate drugs were being adversely affected," Le Perlier went on. "For a full week I attended the state trial of *Pharmacies of the French Republic versus Beljanski*.

"Listening to the final arguments by lawyers for both sides, I fell into shock and became totally discouraged at my lack of condemnatory story material when I heard the prosecutor conclude his case by declaring to the judge that he was ashamed at the circumstances of such a legal action. The prosecutor stated, 'The State is wrongly litigating this case against Dr. Beljanski and instead should be assisting him with the scientific discoveries he is making. Therefore, even as prosecutor against him, I am convinced that the professor's new findings and his other information about degenerative diseases have validity.'" The journalist shook his head at the memory.

Two Years Pass without Negative Statements from Patients

"Despite this great defeat of my mission against Dr. Beljanski, I remained determined to pursue it. I needed to fulfill my obligations to that drug company friend of mine and deliver the story to my newspaper's editors. It was a job I took seriously. I wanted information from anyone who would be critical of the microbiologist.

"I searched for over two years, but I could find absolutely no patient afflicted with some disabling illness and following Beljanski's recommendations who had expressed any bitter or angry feelings about the microbiologist. Sufferers of sickness who took the therapies Beljanski had perfected merely had expressed love, gratefulness, and felt pride in his being a Frenchman. Their feelings result from the great good he has brought to the world.

"For users of his supplements," continued the journalist, "Dr. Beljanski is a medical hero! My conclusion is correct inasmuch as he has prolonged the life of France's most famous man at the time—our republic's president. It's now known that during that same two-year period of my personal journalistic investigations, François Mitterrand, then President of the French Republic, swallowed Beljanski's skillfully prepared plant extracts. He took the herbals to save himself from dying of prostate cancer," Monsieur Le Perlier then confided in me.

"In an important French magazine, *Paris Match*, President Mitterrand responded to the media's criticism of therapy he was receiving for his prostate gland. He assured members of the press and his critics that a medical doctor in Versailles administering prostate gland treatment to him performed a vital service by use of the nonconventional supplements he was dispensing. These products, which he left unnamed, were allowing Mitterrand to survive through his second term of seven years as France's President." However Mitterrand's attending physician, Dr. Gubler, in his book *Le Grand Secret*, explicitly revealed that Mitterrand was indeed benefitting from Beljanski's extracts. For some unknown reason, the French president stopped taking the extracts sometime in 1995. He died January 8, 1996.

Le Perlier's First-Hand Experience

Le Perlier continued, "My newspaper's publisher approached me and declared, 'You really are idiotic in trying for all these many months to write columns entirely negative about Beljanski's work when the President of our French Republic is taking his same supplements. If Beljanski's products are good enough for François Mitterrand, why are they not best for the French people?'

"Of course, *Minute*'s publisher did not know that my friend, the pharmaceutical company executive vice president, had set me on this path of negative investigation," explained the journalist. "I was acting in accordance with the pharmaceutical industry's request to write something critical about Beljanski. How could the publisher comprehend what he cited as my idiocy?

"Subsequently, the entire tone of our newspaper's journalistic approach to this medical story changed to the positive. The task was taken away from me and transferred to other reporters so that a very large feature article about Beljanski was published prominently in *Minute*. In contrast, as its exposé theme," Le Perlier said proudly, "this new feature stated that the true scandal is that Complementary, Alternative and Integrative Medicine (CAIM) is being received by the president of our French Republic as his personal choice for cancer therapy.

"The published feature article in my newspaper unabashedly stated that 'the cancer causation and medication discoverer, Mirko Beljanski, Ph.D., is undergoing constant attack by the Order of French Pharmacists. The druggists' pharmacy association has falsely accused him of making claims for a cancer cure, practicing medicine without a license, and stealing away their pharmaceutical sales.' It was a true exposé piece about greedy druggists rather than describing a charlatan and quack named Beljanski. The value of Beljanski's research was not even questioned. Thus, late in 1995 a positive and uplifting news feature about Dr. Beljanski was printed in *Minute*. The effect was that certain ill people or their loved ones clamored to receive Beljanski's products."

As you can imagine, I was sitting on the edge of my seat at all that Monsieur Le Perlier had related to me. I was beginning to understand that these supplements are currently distributed throughout Europe and in North America as food supplements. Le Perlier also told me that the incidence of specific illnesses in France and some other European countries lessened during the next year of 1996 until, under pressure from the international pharmaceutical industry, the government of France in support of its pharmaceutical industry took direct action to cut off supplies of Beljanski's supplements to the public. As a result, people marched in the streets of Paris and other cities in France to protest the unavailability of the botanicals.

Over time, the political newspaper, *Minute*, fell into a difficult financial situation so that its bills went unpaid. In mid-2000, *Minute* declared bankruptcy and went out of business. During our interview the political journalist explained these economic troubles happened because the Republic of France eliminated the opposition political voice in the newspaper.

Attempting to cope with his newspaper's upsetting financial plight by seeking investors, borrowing money, holding off creditors, conducting negotiations, writing dynamic columns where possible, and doing much more, Monsieur Le Perlier severely felt the stress of his newspaper's difficulty. It seriously weighed on him. He felt acute fatigue which sent him to bed and devastated his production as a reporter.

Simultaneous with the periodical's bankruptcy and his own loss of work, the journalist confronted an ironic twist of fate. He was diagnosed with rectal/colon cancer, which is the fourth most deadly malignancy affecting Frenchmen. There was no doubt about his diagnosis and its severity. Monsieur Le Perlier (M. Le Perlier) found it necessary to call upon his list of valuable contacts with prominent people, including those in medical care. He needed help and called in his markers.

"I visited in Paris with France's national administrator of health who did me a personal favor and referred me to the best and most authoritative expert on colon and rectal cancer in the whole country at that time," Le Perlier told me. "It was medical school professor, Jean Denis, M.D. At his cancer clinic, after my having undergone a massive amount of diagnostic laboratory and clinical evaluations, I asked Dr. Denis to relate the full details of my health. 'Please tell me the truth and pull no punches,' I said to the professor.

"Unceremoniously Dr. Denis sat me down in a chair at his desk and with kindness explained that I had just three more months to live, and they would be absolute hell on earth. He stated, 'Perhaps you will be lucky in that God will take your life sooner so that you won't suffer quite so long.'"

No Standard Medical Treatment Exists

Le Perlier continued, "Dr. Denis explained that there was no medical treatment for me because my rectal/colon cancer was very advanced and had metastasized (when the cancer spreads to new sites in the body) throughout my gut. Any available strong treatment would likely kill me before my cancer totally disabled me," the journalist affirmed. "The doctor added, 'Performing surgery on you will let you survive for just a short time longer, and this you'll be doing while carrying a plastic bag attached to your bowel wall (called a colostomy bag), and the bag will need to be emptied periodically. It would be an awful lifestyle which I do not recommend.'

"At the time I had been living on the outskirts of Paris, and this I needed to change. Therefore, I left my wife and children behind, moved out of our home in my small country town and rented a city apartment on the ground floor. This first floor flat was more appropriate to accommodate my death for its ease of moving my body to the mortuary," Le Perlier explained. "My legal and financial affairs were set into the best possible order manageable. I prepared my mind and emotions to accept death which I anticipated would arrive shortly. My abdomen was giving me severe pain, and I welcomed death so that the pain would stop.

"And then something magnificent happened," Le Perlier said with a broad smile. "A package containing Beljanski's products arrived in the mail, sent by a longtime friend, Serge de Becketch, who was a former writer/editor with me at *Minute*. This fellow journalist had been sick with cancer himself and, having done his share of investigatory journalism on Dr. Mirko Beljanski, he searched for and found the scientist's discoveries which he was convinced would be excellent for me. Then and now de Becketch emphasizes that Beljanski's concept of cancer causation and the botanicals that counteract it had eliminated his own cancer symptoms and preserved his life. He wanted this positive effect for me.

"I just sat and stared at the items de Becketch had sent to me. I made no move to swallow them even over several hours because I truly believed that I was too far gone to benefit from ingesting them," Le Perlier states as he wiped away tears. "I had convinced myself that my body was in the process of producing so many cancer cells that there was no hope. But then I wondered aloud, 'Are you so intent on dying this horrible death that you won't even try using what a friendly fellow worker has mailed to you?'

"Finally my answer was to pop down the doses suggested in Serge de Becketch's accompanying letter to me," Le Perlier says. "By taking the dosages for several weeks, my gut unblocked, my secondary infections of opportunistic organisms such as yeast overgrowth cleared up, my pain went away, and I was able to function and take care of myself. Herpes simplex and yeast infection from *Candida albicans* disappeared; bloody stools stopped coming on with any bowel movement; pain around the rectum discontinued also; and fatigue left me altogether. I could eat real food instead of just sipping shakes and smoothies.

"As I began feeling improved, I was able to take the several more conventional drugs and other products prescribed by various health professionals, including my family doctor, a gastroenterologist, and an additional consulting oncologist. Working synergistically, a combination of Beljanski's and other medications healed my body sufficiently that I could visit the hospital to undergo the recommended exceedingly high-dose radiotherapy," Le Perlier told me. "Of course, before Beljanski's more natural and non-toxic therapies had become available, such radiation treatments would have killed me.

"Not all of Beljanski's supplements had been mailed to me by my friend, Serge de Becketch, but by then I had access to other Beljanski products including a Beljanski-developed form of *Ginkgo biloba* and an herbal regulator of cell enzymes made from fragments of RNA, both of which repair cellular processes even when they are exposed to extreme physiological stresses such as radiation. And I had recently read an article authored by Dr. Mirko Beljanski's wife and former collaborator, Monique Beljanski, which confirms how this very specific preparation of *Ginkgo biloba* works. It helped me exactly as Madame Beljanski (Mme. Beljanski) had written.[7]

"In fact, I have ingested large quantities of all of Dr. Beljanski's supplements and continue to do so even today. Beljanski's discoveries have saved my life, for I am interviewing here with you on September 8, 2003, three years and two months after receiving my diagnosis of colon cancer and the prognosis of only ninety days left to live," affirmed the political journalist. "Today I feel tiptop and remain without any kind of debilitating symptoms."

I am also pleased to note that at the current writing of this book in 2011, M. Le Perlier is still in good health, working and providing for his family.

Who is this Miracle Worker?

I sat astonished at Monsieur Le Perlier's story. If he hadn't told it to me directly, I might have believed it to be a fable. I have published books reporting on effective cancer treatment, but nothing I knew about compared to what this journalist was telling me. I had to find out more, especially after hearing success story after success story from people who had cheated death much like Le Perlier had done. Three years prior to the picnic, I had lost my beloved wife and mother. I knew there were thousands of people dying of cancer right at that very moment. I had to know who this Mirko Beljanski was. From where did he come? How was it that a microbiologist and not a medical doctor had developed such a powerful answer to such a troublesome disease? How did he arrive at this ground-breaking research, and what was it really all about? What *were* these herbal concoctions made of?

1

Mirko Beljanski's Early Years

A dedicated biochemist of humble origin, Dr. Mirko Beljanski was arguably one of the most important scientists of the twentieth century. Graduating with his doctorate in 1951 from the University of Paris, he worked for thirty years as a researcher in molecular biology at the Pasteur Institute, and then spent the remainder of his years tirelessly researching the secrets of DNA and RNA. I believe that Mirko Beljanski, Ph.D., has brought humankind a means of healing beyond all others in the history of medicine. He was a modest man and totally dedicated to improving the health of the human body, but his life could have ended in obscurity, a mere farmer tucked away in the backwaters of northern Serbia. Fortunately for all of us, it did not.

Mirko Beljanski was born in 1923 into a rural family in the northern-most province of Serbia, which was then part of Yugoslavia. His was the large farming village of Turija and its inhabitants were devoted to their corn crops, their pigs, geese, and goats. Mirko Beljanski's father, Milan, worked as a mechanic in the repairing of his neighbors' farm equipment. One of Milan's mechanical talents was the ability to drill fresh water wells for the townspeople, who at the time still had no running water. Electricity came to Turija many years after Mirko had left the place permanently.

The weather in northern Serbia was extremely harsh with freezing cold winters and searing hot summers. Such weather, coupled with the seemingly constant ongoing political struggles that have plagued this region from time immemorial, left his fellow townsfolk to be at times unhopeful about life. His neighbors' negative attitude irritated the boy. He was born with a positive outlook and wanted to do great things in life.

Even at age seven, a thirst for independence and productivity grew in him. Brimming with strong self-discipline, the young Beljanski refused to accept imposed authority or collective discipline. Mirko wanted knowledge, and he recognized that schoolbook learning would allow him to follow his own path out of the limiting Serbian lifestyle and mindset. He put all of his energy into achieving an education. He sought advice from elders and planned with them how he might accomplish his goal.

From his village of six thousand hard-working people, three children were selected for a scholarship to travel to the nearest town twenty-two miles away where there was a small elementary school in combination with a high school. The three Turija students, all thirsty for learning, took a test to see if they were smart enough to warrant their living away from home and attending school. Mirko, eleven years of age, passed and was told he was to leave his family to go live with his Uncle Mitia and his wife in the distant town of Novi-Sad, the capitol of the region. The young Mirko wanted that potential education with all his being. He must have felt ecstatic, knowing he had a chance to make his dream come true.

The boy traveled the required twenty-two miles to Novi-Sad by carriage in the fall of 1934. He resided in his relatives' small, white-cob house consisting of only two clean rooms, one for his uncle and aunt and the other for Mirko and his grandmother. His aunt milked two cows in a small cow shed out back to help the family finances. Mirko's job was to deliver the milk to neighboring houses before the start of each day's classes.

For the first few months in Novi-Sad, the lad found it difficult being apart from his immediate family. Compared to his schoolmates, he felt clumsy and was ashamed that he spoke with a country accent. He was not well travelled; he felt he had poor manners and had no book learning. But what he lacked in sophistication he made up for with an unshakeable will and an uncanny ability to adapt. He was a tireless worker which helped him prevail even when difficult circumstances presented themselves—and they often did in his life.

Once he settled into his schooling, he quickly became well-respected among his teachers. Mirko loved school and was a fast learner. He also got along well with his aunt, uncle, and grandmother. Over the next ten years, Mirko realized that Turija was not a place to which he ever wanted to return. When he returned to visit, he found the time there endless.

In 1942 Mirko successfully passed his Serbian baccalaureate test (the test allowing his graduation from school), and it was just in the nick of time, too. His high school was closed down a couple of days after his graduation because World War II was raging throughout Europe.

In addition to World War II, civil conflict struck Yugoslavia. The entire country was now at war with itself while at the same time trying, and failing, to protect itself from Nazi Germany. Loyalties were divided and tensions ran high. While refusing to be political, different cliques of his friends pushed Mirko to join either with the Yugoslavian partisans, who fought the Germans, or the monarchists who feared communism more than the German invaders and who were attacking the partisans. He held back from joining either side.

Mirko hesitated—he never had been interested in politics—but he finally decided to enlist with the partisans and spent several months traveling clandestinely from farm to farm, relaying messages. He was required to attend political meetings even though he disliked his situation and the way things were being run. His partisan buddies looked with disfavor on Mirko's reserve, especially his lack of enthusiasm regarding some military maneuvers. Additionally, he cherished his freedom of speech and sometimes dared to criticize the "higher ups."

The atmosphere around him was getting tense. By a stroke of good luck, his situation changed. In 1944, Mirko was selected, along with several other Yugoslavian students, to receive a fellowship to continue his scholarship abroad; it was to be either in Moscow or Paris. At a meeting in Belgrade where these promising students assembled to learn the location of their fellowship studies, Mirko found himself in an unlikely group of compatriots: those who did not own a winter coat. Those students who were totally unprepared to face the harsh Moscow winters without warm clothing were automatically assigned to study in Paris, a choice which suited Mirko just fine. Paris had always been his preference. Thus his limited material possessions, along with his humble background, for once helped give him a great opportunity. And so it was that on a rainy day in the autumn of 1945, Mirko Beljanski arrived on the streets of Paris.

Mirko, the Student

Taking shelter in local student hostels, young Mirko Beljanski settled into a scholar's life in Paris. Registration for college took place at the Sorbonne, where Mirko intended to obtain his doctoral degree in science. To participate in classes, he was required to learn French and to speak and read it fluently. Money was scarce; there was barely enough earned cash to rent a room, eat one good meal a day, and buy books. While he did experience his first romances, the young man preferred to remain on his own in order to fully dedicate himself to work in the sciences. Mirko had a great love of learning. He did well in chemistry but found his passion in biology.

He completed his undergraduate degree in 1947, intending to start work on his doctoral thesis right away. Before starting as a graduate student, however, a letter arrived from Mirko's mother. She wrote him asking that he return home. She needed Mirko to come home and help the family by resuming work as a farmer. His mother didn't, and I'm sure couldn't, understand what was important to her son. To her, the income he could gain from milking a few more cows far outweighed any book learning. But Mirko had other ideas. He knew he wanted to be a scientist and did not wish to leave school, but since his academic scholarship had run out and after a brief stint at the Biology Institute on Pierre Curie Street in Paris, he decided to fulfill his obligation to return to his family and his Yugoslavian village.

The budding scientist was never destined to return to farm life. Before he returned home, a new opportunity presented itself. He was able to assist with the Beljanski family's finances by working for six months in a laboratory in Yugoslavia's major city, Belgrade. Then luck smiled on him again. He received another Sorbonne scholarship which allowed him to return to Paris. This good fortune was followed quickly by an International Affairs academic scholarship which allowed him to start his doctoral thesis. He joined the Pasteur Institute, and Professor Michel Macheboeuf, Ph.D., became Beljanski's supervisor for his doctoral thesis. Reports suggest that the director was impressed with the young, hard-working student. The elder scientist knew he needed a meticulous researcher to carry on the difficult work he was doing on antibiotics. Beljanski had an affinity for biology already, so we can only assume he took up the work his mentor offered to him with gusto.

Initial Research of the Young Biochemist

Dr. Macheboeuf was head of the investigative laboratory in the Department of Cellular Biology at the Pasteur Institute. Beljanski began his student training under the direct supervision of this highly intelligent, empathetic, and kind professor of biochemistry. In 1948, Dr. Macheboeuf suggested that his student investigate the origin of bacterial resistance against various antibiotics for his Ph.D. thesis. At the time, streptomycin, a potent killer of pathological organisms (commonly called pathogens), was the dramatic new antibiotic coming out of World War II and was just beginning to be used by medical consumers.

As one of its most vital applications, streptomycin has been among the most effective antibiotics for putting active pulmonary tuberculosis into remission or even curing it. But the natural resistance of tubercle bacilli (the bacteria that causes tuberculosis) sometimes leaves behind thousands of organisms totally unaffected by streptomycin; consequently, the antibiotic often must be combined and administered with another antibiotic, thus allowing different mechanisms of action to attack the tuberculosis infection.

This sort of problem occupied Beljanski's mental efforts and laboratory skills during the four years that he worked toward his doctorate, which he acquired in 1951. The young biochemical researcher carried out Professor Macheboeuf's recommendations and went even further. He proved that several antibiotics used were capable of inducing modifications in RNA. (RNA is one of three major components essential for all known life forms, along with DNA and proteins).

His laboratory notes record that several species of streptomycin-resistant mutant bacteria tend to accumulate certain types of RNA during a given period. Numerous published papers came out of his research not only on streptomycin but also on other antibiotics-resistant organisms.[8]

Upon gaining his doctoral degree in molecular biology, which is a sub-science of biochemistry concerned with understanding interactions between the various systems of a cell, Mirko Beljanski was drawn to the then new profession of microbiology—the study of even smaller living units, primarily bacteria, viruses, and fungi. His preliminary studies allowed him to select the methods of analysis which were to become essential in his subsequent research.

Once again he conferred with his mentor, Professor Macheboeuf. Macheboeuf recognized Beljanski's courage, imagination, and persistent nature; he understood how Mirko was quite different from the other young graduates. In place of philosophizing or intellectualizing, the new Ph.D. preferred working alone, driven by an inner need to sculpt and establish his own beliefs and find his own truths. Beljanski found great rapport with Macheboeuf and was overjoyed to share the byline with him on four published scientific papers or any other kind of work under his mentor's direct supervision.[9]

From the beginning of his research career, Mirko Beljanski was a man connected to experimentation, from his laboratory animals to his lab benches where various microscopes, test tubes, Bunsen burners, and beakers were strewn about ready for use.

Starting a New Life

In 1951 as Mirko completed his Ph.D. in biochemistry, he also had other things on his mind. With a new doctoral diploma and a French paycheck to take home, he decided to propose marriage to the French girl he had been dating, the young and beautiful Mademoiselle Monique Lucas. Very much in love, she accepted and the couple was married in Yugoslavia.

The bride's middle-income French parents set them up in a pretty little apartment on a Paris back street, not too far from the Pasteur Institute. Mirko wanted his young wife to be by his side as much as possible, so he persuaded the bride to enroll in a school for laboratory and bacteriology technicians. Monique passed the two-year course with honors. She became newly certified as a laboratory assistant in Professor Michel Macheboeuf's laboratory and entered the CNRS, the French National Center for Scientific Research. CNRS has been a long-time research partner of the Pasteur Institute and is now a government-funded research organization under the administrative authority of France's Ministry of Research. That same year, Mirko also joined the CNRS as a researcher.

That first working arrangement for them was the beginning of over a quarter-century of joint research undertakings. Mutual respect for each other lasted for the rest of their lives, united in work that was pure joy, a symbol of their togetherness, and the source of many intellectual adventures.

At the Pasteur, Beljanski continued his investigations into antibiotics and genetics. The newlyweds worked intensively on experiments involving bacterial resistance to antibiotics. They cooperated well together as laboratory colleagues. Beljanski was a man possessed, and during several interviews with Monique, she recounted to me some of their more interesting adventures. Once, Mirko awoke Monique at 3:00 a.m., dragged her out of bed and into the cool Paris streets so that they could dig some

Petri dishes out of the laboratory garbage at the Pasteur Institute. They had thrown them away the day before because they thought the experiment in those dishes had failed. But in the middle of the night, Mirko wondered if all of the bacterial colonies in this particular lab test could have, in fact, mutated instead of only making the expected isolated, random changes. Monique and Mirko climbed the fences surrounding the Institute, ran to the trash bins in order to beat the garbage collector, and found that, in fact, every cell had mutated. These petri dishes became important to later research because Mirko was able to turn back the same type of mutations with a specific chemical taken from blood. Ultimately, all this (and much more) led Beljanski down the research path to his discoveries of cancerous DNA.

Here again was another gigantic "what if" in the story of his amazing discoveries. What if Beljanski had *not* awoken that early morning years ago and insisted his wife accompany him on his trash-sifting adventure? He might have found a path to his ground-breaking research another way, but he might not have, just as he could have elected to stay on the farm and raise geese and pigs instead of giving the world a potentially viable way to handle one of the most deadly and feared diseases on the planet.

Paradise Lost

Beljanski was motivated purely by science. As a microbiologist, he wanted to use his abilities and knowledge to work to better the lives of his fellow human beings. He had a very simple yet systematic way of going about solving any problem with which he was faced:

first—sifting through various biochemical experimental projects

second—setting up and completing the inevitable next experiment

third—discovering from research the biological questions needing answers.

Underlying it all was a commitment to constant, meticulous research. Hard work never discouraged Mirko. The two or three technicians working with him at their laboratory benches ran around day and night, each technician performing a vital operation in the piece of work being studied. This buzz of activity irritated his colleagues who scoffed at it, confusing passion for one's work with opportunism.

Mirko Beljanski was not an opportunist. Rather, he was a man totally consumed by his research endeavors. He was driven to understand nature and to make an original contribution for the benefit of humankind, leaving a positive mark by advancing his ideas. Most demanding of himself, he also demanded a great deal from his team members. He was often short on patience while rushing toward the completion of a goal.

Because he did not take the time to gossip with colleagues who seemed to discuss at length how to recreate the world, Mirko made almost no friends among them. His lack of availability due to his devotion to his work was misunderstood. Instead, his colleagues interpreted Mirko's absence as aloofness or pretension.

While their assessment was incorrect, it is true that Mirko was not very approachable. From his Yugoslavian peasant origins, he retained a concrete mentality and did not enjoy the theorizing so beloved by French intellectuals. For such aloof-like behavior, Mirko Beljanski was rejected by coworkers, and this resulted in the failure of his colleagues to afford him the appropriate degree of recognition he deserved.

In 1952, Mirko's much loved mentor, Michel Macheboeuf, Ph.D., chief of his Pasteur Institute department, passed away suddenly. Dr. Macheboeuf had been exposed to poisonous gas during World War I, which resulted in chronic lung damage. From time to time, he had experienced debilitating episodes involving one of the lobes of his lungs. The lung's weakness eventually led to Macheboeuf developing a bronchial lung cancer, which finally killed him during the summer of 1952.

To replace Macheboeuf as director of the Department of Cellular Biochemistry, the Pasteur's governing board named Jacques Monod,

Ph.D. Mirko, Monique, and other researchers who had worked for the late Macheboeuf, were integrated into Dr. Monod's expanded team of scientists. But there was a problem: Jacques Monod and Mirko Beljanski didn't like each other at all.

The conflict between them was ongoing. Very aware of his own personal image, Monod was not interested in Mirko's investigatory strengths and did not appreciate the researcher's straightforwardness. Simultaneously, Mirko failed to take into account the media savvy of his new boss, whom he believed to be more excited by the limelight of public relations than by the study of science. These two strong and opposing egos were simply not made for mutual cooperation, and they often clashed. Shortly after he had been named as head of the Department of Cellular Biochemistry, Monod asked Beljanski, as they passed each other in the hall, "What do you think? Should I accept the offer to head our department?"

Jacques Monod craved praise and approval from everyone at the Pasteur. Satisfaction for his ego was everything for Dr. Monod. Dr. Beljanski did nothing to feed that satisfaction. He replied to his new boss, "But you already have accepted the position, so why ask my opinion?"

At first shocked by the answer to his question, Monod turned off all style and charm and went on his way without comment. However, he did not let it rest. The new director related the occurrence between him and Beljanski to his colleagues, and they let it be known that Monod hated Beljanski all the more for his undiplomatic response and would refuse him his scientific backing.

Any observer would judge that these were two temperaments that only the love of science could bring together, but their conceptions of science had vastly different values. The boss wanted it to service him in his career; the worker wanted to dedicate his life to its service. From the first moments of their first meeting, any civil dialogue between them became practically impossible.

Alleviating the Tension

Since Monod thrived exceedingly well as a scientist-politician-publicist with lots of connections to the political, commercial, and international community, greater amounts of budget money came along with his appointment as department head. He set about using the new money to transform and modernize the old laboratory facilities.

Structural plans were drawn up for the department, contractors were hired, and the staff was then exposed to many months of building reconstruction. Each day they faced dust, debris, construction noise, and supply shortages. Worthwhile work became impossible for everyone. The scientists in the cellular biochemistry department left for other laboratories in Europe, Canada, Australia, or the U.S.

Early in 1956, Beljanski was offered a two-year scholarship at New York University (NYU) to undertake research with Severo Ochoa, Ph.D. Because the personality conflict had not improved between Dr. Beljanski and Dr. Monod, acceptance of Dr. Ochoa's invitation was encouraged by Director Monod. He preferred Mirko and Monique to be gone from the Pasteur Institute for as long as possible—perhaps permanently.

The early to mid-1950s was a very exciting time for biologists and biochemists. The structure of DNA (which will be explained later) was discovered in 1953 and everyone, it seemed, turned their attention to this breakthrough. Many notions that today are routinely taught were as yet unknown at that time. The greatest challenge for biochemists and/or biologists in those years of the 1950s was mapping the genetic code. Such mapping keenly interested both Dr. Ochoa and Dr. Beljanski, and part of that process was uncovering the mechanisms that had to do with protein synthesis.

Protein synthesis is an exceedingly important but very complex chemical process, for it creates protein, which is the main building block of cell structure. During that period, very little was understood about the functioning of protein synthesis, and many biochemists devoted much of their time researching the hidden mechanisms through which cells create proteins. Drs. Ochoa and Beljanski were no different. For two years Beljanski, with his wife always at his side, performed experiments to understand how amino acids are selected during the natural process of combining with each other to become peptides. Amino acids are the basic unit or building blocks of proteins and when linked together in chains form a polypeptide. When the amino acids from different parts of the chain interact with each other, the polypeptide chain takes on a unique shape forming a protein.

It was an extremely difficult task to determine what factors governed specific combinations of amino acids and/or peptides during protein synthesis, but it was a job that Professor Ochoa asked his new associate to accept. Mirko did so with enthusiasm. Together they conducted experiments to incorporate radioactive amino acids into the systems of living organisms. Then they reported their observations. As co-investigators and co-authors they eventually published three scientific papers together.[10]

Dr. Ochoa was a charming, courteous, refined man and always pleasant. The three scientists respected each other and got along exceedingly well. Ochoa appreciated the enthusiasm the two young French visitors brought to their work. As a result of his work with RNA and its relationship to peptides in protein synthesis, Mirko Beljanski was recognized by his colleagues. He received the 1960 Charles-Leopold Mayer Prize from the French Academy of Sciences for valuable work performed during the preceding years in molecular biology. Dr. Ochoa himself was looking for an enzyme that he eventually found and called *polynucleotide phosphorylase* (PNPase). Ochoa went on to show that this enzyme was capable of synthesizing RNAs in a test tube. It was for these discoveries in biochemistry that he later became famous (having received a Nobel Prize in 1959), and the two Beljanskis used his findings to perfect their own experiments.

The time spent by Ochoa and Beljanski researching in areas of common interest was quite productive. They recorded a body of knowledge which the world-wide scientific community still utilizes. They set precedents which have not been overturned.

Back to Paris

During the summer of 1956, Monique was expecting the young couple's first child, Sylvie. While the mother-to-be found herself forced to remain away from working at NYU, Mirko continued to experience satisfaction and success with his biochemical investigations in the Ochoa laboratory. After a year of working together, Dr. Ochoa suggested that Mirko settle in the U.S. permanently and become an American. But the Beljanskis felt they belonged back in France. They wanted to raise their children there, and Mirko was very attached to Monique's parents. In 1958, when Monique found that she was expecting their second child, Boris, the couple decided that they wanted their baby to be born and their children raised in France. Therefore at the end of Mirko's two-year fellowship, the family returned to France.

Little did they realize just how important their decision to return home would prove to be. Due to differences in the way research is financed in the United States as compared to France, it seems unlikely that Mirko's exhaustive and complex investigations could have been accomplished in the United States at all.

In France, a CNRS researcher is a bit like a civil servant: he has job security and salary security which allows him to carry out in-depth research without the constraints of having to first prove its profitability. In contrast, the American system of scientific research requires an investigator to dedicate a significant part of his time to obtaining funding each year. This creates the incentive for rapid results but does not allow the researcher a period of time for reflection. That ability to reflect on research results was key for Beljanski.

After two years of working at NYU, Dr. Beljanski and his wife returned to resume work in the newly constructed Pasteur Institute facilities. While the couple was glad to be back home in France, they had little enthusiasm about coming back to Monod's department.

On his return, Beljanski wished to pursue the investigations he had begun in the United States, while Monod wanted him to study a particular enzyme, a biochemical subject to which his laboratory was dedicated because it had to do with the genetic aspect of DNA. Beljanski refused because his findings were all in contradiction with such a scheme.

Upset at hearing Beljanski's refusal to investigate the enzyme in question, Dr. Monod, in a fit of anger, declared to Beljanski, "But everyone works on my ideas!"

Mirko responded without hesitation, "Exactly! That's already plenty of people, so let me go my own way!"

Mirko and Monique stood their ground, and Monod finally allowed the two Beljanskis to do what they wanted at their laboratory bench; however, from that day forward he no longer took any interest in the discoveries the Beljanskis were making.

Monod was a difficult yet brilliant man. A testimony to Monod's brilliance came in 1965 when he shared the Nobel Prize in Physiology or Medicine with François Jacob, Ph.D., and André Lwoff, Ph.D., for work concerning the control of the genetic expression in DNA (the part of DNA that has to do with the pattern of physical characteristics of the human body).

The ideas of Monod and Beljanski were in conflict over whether changes in DNA came only from mutations (alterations in the primary structure of the DNA), or whether, as Beljanski asserted, without contradicting the role of mutations, the environment could influence DNA functioning in ways other than through mutation.

Beljanski's opinion was that environmental substances could interfere with the ability of DNA to replicate itself properly which would influence the functioning of DNA but not cause mutation; Monod did not believe this was so. Beljanski also thought, in contrast to Monod, that RNA could influence the functioning of DNA in various ways, rather than just DNA affecting the functioning of RNA. At that time, the idea of influencing DNA other than through mutations was considered to be an insult to the dogma of DNA supremacy, a dogma which was championed by Monod.

Nowadays, many scientists are aware of the response a cell's substances have to its surrounding. Yet Mirko Beljanski was one of the first, if not *the* first, to give a molecular definition and concrete examples of the role the environment plays in DNA functioning improperly and that phenomena's relationship to cancer causation.

Monod concepts, however, were championed by the scientific community around the world and prejudiced the minds of scientists for a full generation after he published his findings. Jacques Monod was also the political darling of the French nation, especially after he brought the Nobel Prize to France; what he declared as truth became the accepted dogma for the nation. Scientifically, Beljanski and his ideas were at complete odds with Monod, a conflict that would haunt Beljanski for the remainder of his life.

The discord between the scientific ideas of Dr. Monod and Dr. Beljanski was not helped by the constant strife created by the deep-seated personality clash between the two men. As Monique recounted during our New York City meeting on Thursday, June 24, 2005, "Mirko would meditate about his work and was never quick to jump to conclusions, as do some brilliant people. Jacques Monod was brilliant, but tended to be closed to ideas that differed from his own. My husband was totally different from him. Their personalities clashed often. Monod was distrustful of Mirko; Mirko felt impatient with Monod's inflated ego."

Monique spoke about her husband in a frank and candid way; she used a respectful tone of voice and a mildness of expression as if almost in awe. She continued, "Mirko Beljanski hated the word *genius*, and denied the term for himself. He declared instead, 'I am no genius and hardly possess much intelligence. If I find success from my investigations, it's because I am a hard worker, stay persistent in my efforts, and possess a free mind that remains open to ideas no matter how outlandish they may seem.'"

Mirko was in no way bothered by the boss' disinterest in or contempt for his work simply because our dauntless researcher preferred to work alone. Although independent, he developed his convictions from observations he made during his experiments, while drawing hypotheses and theories to explain such observations.

Dr. Beljanski continued to work at the Pasteur Institute for almost twenty more years under Monod as it had the facilities and tools necessary for studying enzymes, nucleic acids, plants and animals. The latter was particularly important since Mirko wanted his results to be applicable to the general laws of the living world. In those twenty years, no matter what else occurred between the two rivals, Beljanski's research work at the Pasteur netted great benefits for the health of all humankind. Concepts of disease development evolved and therapies to reverse such diseases resulted from these efforts. Eventually people with various illnesses, especially those involving cancer, found that this humble biochemist had much to offer them.

2
Destabilized DNA:
Cancer Lies in the Structure of DNA

Before the advent of antibiotics, strep infection was a major killer of infants; staph infection claimed the lives of 80 percent of those whose wounds were infected with it, and anyone who came down with tuberculosis or pneumonia basically had their death certificates handed to them. These were diseases that no one knew how to fight until Alexander Fleming, a bacteriologist working at St. Mary's hospital in London, found that a mold on a discarded culture plate had somehow killed the *staphylococci* bacteria that had been on the same plate. It was 1928 and, of course, the mold in question was penicillin.[11] Suddenly diseases considered deadly were now curable, and the world rejoiced.

Today cancer, seconded only by AIDS, has become the most dreaded of modern diseases for the same simple reason pneumonia was so feared less than a hundred years ago. It appears to be very difficult to cure.

Throughout the forty years that Dr. Mirko Beljanski dedicated to researching DNA and RNA in the human cell, he not only revealed the secrets of what happens to the DNA in a cell that has been affected by a carcinogen, but he discovered a way to counteract the consequences of the cancerous DNA cell. In so doing, he offered a natural alternative to harsh chemical treatments. While cancer will always be potentially deadly, it doesn't have to be so overwhelmingly frightening.

To understand how important Beljanski's findings are to the problem of cancer, we have to first understand a little about the most fundamental parts of a cell. Biology lesson number one is that there are two acids in the center, or nucleus, of a cell. These are called nucleic acids and are better known by the terms DNA (Deoxyribonucleic Acid) and RNA (Ribonucleic Acid). In chapter 4, I will talk about the breakthrough discoveries Dr. Beljanski developed to handle cancer at the DNA level. But in order to appreciate the enormous importance of his findings, it is first necessary to delve into the discoveries he made about the structure of DNA and why, when that structure starts replicating out of control, you develop cancer.

To comprehend cancerous DNA, let us first define cancer. "Cancer" is the name given to that class of diseases in which the body's cells become abnormal, then continue to subdivide, and replicate themselves in the abnormal state indefinitely. Healthy cells are preprogrammed to die at a certain point. This preprogrammed cell death present in healthy cells, called apoptosis, somehow gets shut off in a cancer cell. These rogue cells multiply and multiply, forming a tumor which crowds out the healthy cells in whatever body tissue it's formed. Eventually these cancerous cells metastasize, which means the cancer spreads and forms more tumors in other parts of the body.

It's no wonder cancer is such a feared disease. It isn't an infection, which means that something like bacteria has invaded the cells. You can kill bacteria. But how do you regulate cells that grow with no control, can spread quickly to other parts of the body, and seem to defy all restrictive treatment that modern medicine throws at them? To compound the problem, there are over one hundred different types of cancer, and not all cancer cells behave the same.

The Form and Function of DNA

All through the late 1950s, the scientific world was abuzz with the discoveries of the three biochemists/microbiologists credited with uncovering the structure of DNA. James Watson, Ph.D., Francis Crick, Ph.D., and Maurice Wilkins, Ph.D., building on the X-ray images created by radiation expert Rosalind Franklin, Ph.D., unveiled the power and beauty of DNA. In 1962 Watson, Crick, and Wilkins, with their specialties in the physical sciences (biology, chemistry, and physics), were awarded the Nobel Prize in Physiology or Medicine for their 1953 discovery. Unfortunately, Dr. Franklin was not included in this group because the Nobel is only awarded to a maximum of three scientists, and they have to be living. Dr. Franklin, who had discovered the X-ray images of DNA first, had died of radiation poisoning previous to the 1962 award. There is some evidence that her work is not fully recognized or acknowledged, but whatever the case, these four scientists gave the world one of the most important scientific discoveries in the history of humankind.

The actual identification of DNA is attributed to a scientist named Avery in 1944, but even earlier investigations going back to the turn of the twentieth century were concerned with DNA as genetic material (Boveri from 1902 to 1914 and Sutton in 1903). The major break-through Drs. Watson, Crick, and Wilkins found was that the long strands of DNA sitting in the center of the cell, its nucleus, are structured in a formation that looks like a spiraling ladder. That is, of course, the double helix, and it's called that because a helix could be considered as a spiral or anything twisted. A double helix is simply two such spirals twisted together. Here you can see the shape of the spiraling ladder.

The DNA contains all the information needed to make and control every cell within a living organism. In a way it is wonderfully simple. The structure of the double helix includes both the sides and the rungs of the ladder. The *sides* of the ladder are made up of a combination of the most fundamental elements in nature: carbon, hydrogen, oxygen, nitrogen, and phosphorus. These elements combine to form sugar phosphates, but they

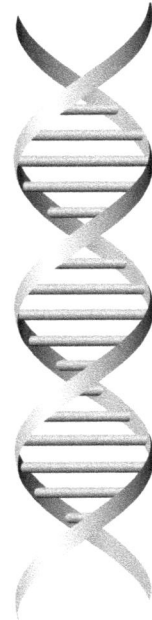

THE DNA DOUBLE HELIX

Figure 1

53

are not the important part of the ladder for our purposes.

The *rungs* of the DNA ladder are made up of four specific nitrogen- containing molecules that are also known as the nitrogenous base, or "bases" of DNA. These four molecules are thymine (T), adenine (A), cytosine (C), and guanine (G). These bases always come in pairs. Thymine (T) will only pair with adenine (A) (also called the "pyrimidine" base pair). Cytosine (C) will only pair with guanine (G) (also called the "purine" base pair). Each pair together is called a base pair, and it doesn't matter in what order the molecules in the base pair are placed. Sometimes it's TA; sometimes, AT. Sometimes it's CG; sometimes, GC.

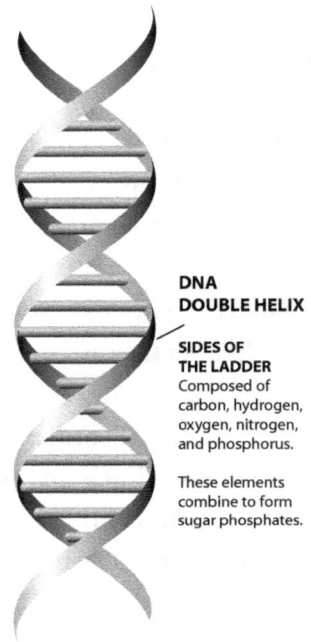

DNA DOUBLE HELIX

SIDES OF THE LADDER
Composed of carbon, hydrogen, oxygen, nitrogen, and phosphorus.

These elements combine to form sugar phosphates.

Figure 2

The Two Functions of DNA

DNA is probably the most vital or consequential molecule for life, since it carries instructions for the maintenance of our bodies. DNA has two main functions:

1. Genetic—DNA carries instructions for the maintenance of a given species through the nature and the positioning of its genes. It does this by permitting specific RNA molecules to "read" the message contained in the genes

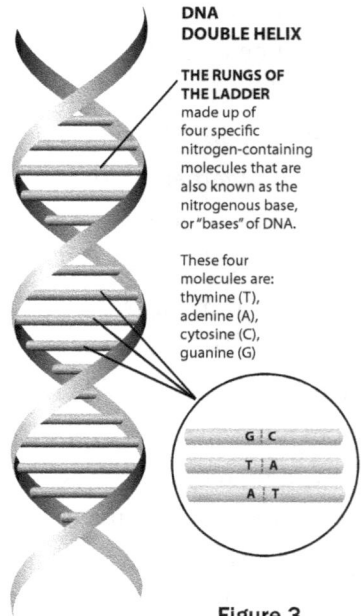

DNA DOUBLE HELIX

THE RUNGS OF THE LADDER
made up of four specific nitrogen-containing molecules that are also known as the nitrogenous base, or "bases" of DNA.

These four molecules are: thymine (T), adenine (A), cytosine (C), guanine (G)

G : C
T : A
A : T

Figure 3

and then, through a series of steps, produce specific proteins to help manage the organism (this is the protein synthesis I briefly outlined in chapter 1). Tens of thousands of different human gene-types exist, with most geneticists putting the total number of genes carried by our chromosomes at approximately one hundred thousand.[12]

2. Self-Replicating—DNA assures self-replication and duplication, which is the first step in cell multiplication. The DNA replicates itself, causing the cell to grow twice its size. Once the cell has replicated itself in its entirety, the cell then divides into two. This process happens trillions of times a day in our bodies.[13] (See Figure 8 on page 62 for a full explanation of DNA replication).

In terms of genetics, the pairing of the bases together are called genes, and they are the basis of all the information that is carried in your body. Knowing this is important simply because your genes govern all of your physical appearance—eye color, hair color, height, sex—every property that has to do with the physical aspect of our bodies. Even more amazing is that most of the body's cells contain a complete sample of our DNA. If you watch any crime scene show on T.V., you're familiar with the importance of DNA as a unique marker for any one person.

Self-replication, the duplication of the DNA molecule, is crucial for the stability and durability of the species because that is how cells produce more cells which cause life to continue.

The Importance of Structure

Indeed, DNA has proven itself to be the most significant molecule in the creation of life. It is closer to perfection than anything else created by nature, God, or man. According to Monod and his loyal followers, it would almost be a sin to believe otherwise. But privileging the importance of the genetic aspects of DNA disallows the importance of its structure. With the discovery of the double helix of DNA, however, the microscopic world of a cell's nucleus was opened up, and the possibilities it presented in terms of understanding disease and, more importantly, how to cure or even prevent diseases in the first place were vast.

Rather than make assumptions over the course of his professional life researching DNA, enzymes, and RNA, Dr. Beljanski studied all aspects of pathology and chose instead to test and observe abnormalities first hand. His findings were almost always original and illuminating. He was a genuine investigator, concerned with using the work he did at his laboratory bench, rather than relying on published books and journals for his information, to help the betterment of humankind.

It was not the genetic aspect of DNA (the part that controls the pattern of physical characteristics of a human body) that ultimately caught Beljanski's attention. Rather it was the structure itself, the way that the DNA molecule was put together in its double helix formation that fascinated the researcher.

More to the point, Beljanski's meticulous original research led him to conclude in the late 1980s that the major source of cancerous cell behavior is caused by *structural corruption* of the DNA.

This conclusion is revolutionary for one simple reason: once DNA became the element of the cell to study, the scientific world focused on the mechanism of gene *mutation* as the basis for cancer from the late 1950s onward. Because in part to scientists like Monod, the prevailing idea of cancer is that it is caused by genetic mutations in the cellular DNA.

When DNA splits and copies itself, it can undergo mutations, alterations, and breakages or other modifications in its structure, all of which lead to alterations in the cell. A mutation is a genetic change that is inherited by all the offspring of the original cell in which the mutation occurred. Luckily, there are systems in our body able to repair these mutations, but sometimes they do not or cannot repair the problem.

A cell or an organism affected by a mutation is described as a mutant. Something that causes mutation in a cell is called a mutagen. The effects of many mutations are well known and those that affect our physical appearance may be striking, as in the case when two fingers are fused together when a baby is born. The most common mutation we're familiar with is Down's syndrome. Mutations happen all the time in a cell, but our cells are programmed to repair the defect and oftentimes the mutation remains harmless even if it isn't corrected.

The mutational theory of cancer basically says that when mutations occur in genes that tell the cell to divide, regulation of this process may be lost and the cells may continue to divide and multiply out of control.[14] Unregulated cell division is a characteristic of cancer-cell growth. That is why the search for significant mutations has long been considered the priority issue in cancer research and why studies of DNA and cancer have focused on the genetic aspect of DNA.

Beljanski was well aware of the fact that cancer sometimes develops from mutations that occur in the DNA. However, he found through hundreds of hours of painstaking research that cancer can be caused by environmental carcinogens (substances that cause cancer) that don't necessarily act as mutagens. He discovered that many carcinogens induce physical structural (not genetic) changes in the DNA, and in order to understand what *that* means, we need to turn now to biology lesson number two on DNA, its primary and secondary structures, and how it replicates.

DNA Replication

As I noted above, when a cell replicates, it allows life to continue. When a cell replicates out of control, it is cancerous. The self-replication of DNA happens at the structural level, and there is a primary and a secondary part to that structure.

The sugar-phosphate side of the DNA ladder is bonded covalently to one of the groups of the two pairs of

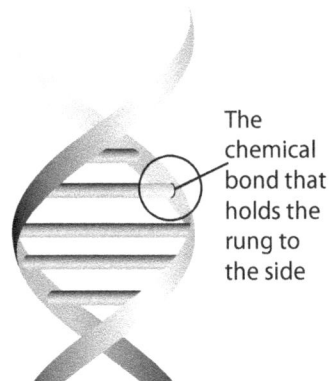

The chemical bond that holds the rung to the side

Figure 4: Covalent Bond

bases, or rungs, of the ladder (the TA/AT or CG/GC combinations). Covalent bonds hold the rungs to the sides in a chemical bond formed by the sharing of electrons (electron being the particle of an atom that is negatively charged). Covalent bonds are very strong because the negative particles of one molecule bond together with the positive particles of another molecule, thereby creating a stable balance of positive and negative forces.

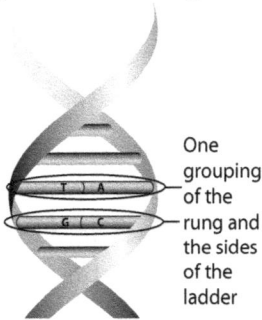

Figure 5: Nucleotide

One grouping of the rung and the sides of the ladder

Together, the sugar-phosphate sides and the nitrogenous bases or rungs of the ladder are called a nucleotide. The nucleotides in the double chain are considered the *primary structure* of the helix. Nucleotides are bound together in long chains, and while the structure of this is in fact quite complicated, what matters for our discussion here is mutations are any alteration of the primary molecular structure of DNA (most often when there is an unplanned change in one base to another).

The *secondary structure* of the DNA molecule is the middle part of the rung of the ladder. The two base pairs are held together by a hydrogen bond. Hydrogen bonds are much weaker than the covalent bonds that hold the rungs to the sides of the ladder. This secondary structure of DNA is where Dr. Beljanski focused much of his attention because of what happens to that hydrogen bond in cancerous DNA.

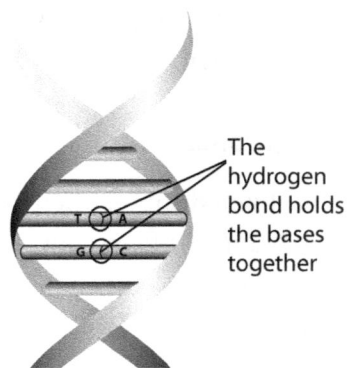

The hydrogen bond holds the bases together

Figure 6: Secondary Structure

The bases or rungs of the ladder held together by the hydrogen bonds I just mentioned act like the teeth of a zipper. When the DNA molecule is zipped up with all its hydrogen bonds intact, it is a very stable and unshakable molecule. It is hard to mess with it. But DNA is constantly replicating itself to make new cells in the body. To do that, it has to unzip itself, and that's where all the trouble lies.

Cells divide and replicate trillions of times in our body every day. It's a normal process. It starts with the DNA making a copy of itself. Then the rest of the cell copies its parts. When the copy is complete, it splits off from the parent cell. The copied cell is then "all of a piece," ready and able to do whatever job it's meant to do.

DNA replication, the heart of cell replication, is really an enigma. It is so small you have to use special microscopes to view it, but it is also unimaginably large in scope. It takes place at rates between fifty nucleotides per second in mammals to five hundred nucleotides per second in bacteria. To give you a sense of the scope of the amount of replication that is taking place in your body right now, do some simple math. Fifty nucleotides replicating per second means that *one* cell is duplicating itself around 4.3 million times a day. There is no consensus on how many cells are in a human body, but estimates range from 50 to 100 *trillion* (a trillion is a million million of something. It is almost impossible to conceive of such a large number). Another way to put it— the nucleotides in your cells reproduce more times in one hour than there are dollars missing in the U.S.'s national current deficit of fourteen trillion dollars. And that's just in a healthy cell. Cancer cells divide and replicate themselves in an out-of-control fashion—far faster than a healthy cell.

How DNA Recreates Itself by Replication

Like every form of life, individual cells have a lifespan. Rather than measure lifespan as a length of time, the lifespan of a cell is measured by how many times it can replicate itself. An average number of replications of cells observed in laboratory experiments is fifty but is theorized to be at a maximum of eighty. When a cell is no longer able to replicate, apoptosis (self-induced cell death) is the result. Self-induced cell death is exceedingly important for the overall health of body tissues. Without apoptosis, every newborn organism would otherwise in reality be just one ongoing cancer with its physiological systems overrun by excessive numbers of growing cells.

Figure 7 shows DNA replication—the recreations of itself again and again. There are a series of steps that it must go through:

1. The top of the illustration shows a "parental" DNA molecule. The rungs of the parental DNA (the bases bound together with a hydrogen bond) break apart and the sides of the ladder break off (the zipper unzips itself). The parent molecule floats off and the open-sided rungs of the ladder are ready to replicate.

2. Open, unbonded bases can now be acted upon by the DNA polymerase, the crucial enzyme that literally makes a new copy of these open, unbonded bases (the open half of the ladder). The copy the DNA polymerase makes is actually complementary to the existing half. If you look at the illustration, you will notice that the side of the ladder that's from the parent DNA molecule has the A, the T, the C, and the G waiting for their proper mates. The DNA polymerase makes a strand that has the corresponding T, A, G, C bases ready to fuse with the existing half.

3. The existing half of the ladder then fuses with the replicated, complimentary half because the hydrogen bonds between the bases reform. The process continues until two identical molecules of DNA have been formed. This happens twice, once for each side of the ladder that was split from the parent DNA molecule. (One zipper is now two and both are zipped up.) In a healthy cell, this process continues in each cell until the cell reaches its maximum number of times it can divide, and its preprogrammed death, apoptosis, occurs.

Figure 7: DNA Replication

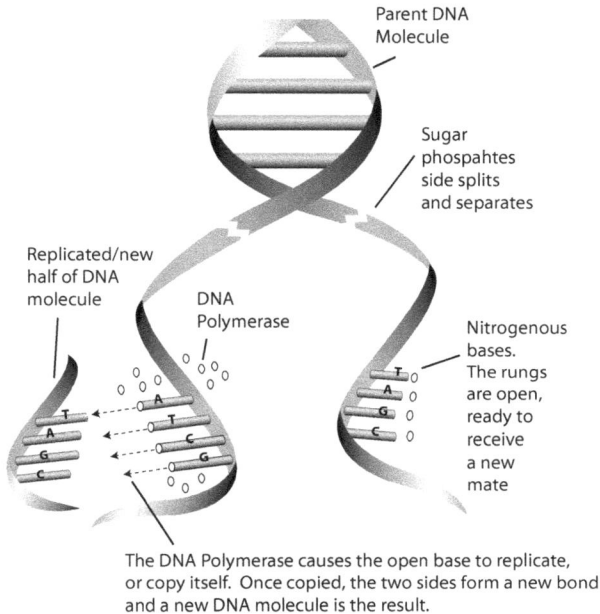

The DNA Polymerase causes the open base to replicate, or copy itself. Once copied, the two sides form a new bond and a new DNA molecule is the result.

This is a remarkably efficient system, and in a perfectly healthy body it runs along smoothly. However, the two strands are bound together by hydrogen bonds whose opening and closing are susceptible to internal and external influences. When the hydrogen bonds of the base pairs fail to rezip, the message that DNA delivers may be dramatically modified. The hydrogen bonding is disrupted by many types of molecules that come from both inside the body and from outside substances such as pollutants that the body absorbs through air, food, water, or even through the skin. These modifications lead to the replication process malfunctioning, which brings on the appearance of various serious diseases such as cancer. It is this malfunctioning that Dr. Beljanski discovered and named DNA destabilization.

DNA Destabilization

DNA interacts with many types of molecules, and these interactions may affect the fate of the cell. DNA initiates the production of other cells, so ensuring the integrity of the DNA is of prime importance in maintaining the structural integrity of cells.

Structural integrity, however, can be compromised by damage either to the primary structure (the order and nature of the base pairs) or the secondary structure (the hydrogen bonding of the base pairs). To reiterate an important point I made above, primary structural damage is usually caused by a mutation of a base or the activation or deactivation of a base by its binding to another molecule. This is the prevailing idea of what happens to the DNA in a cancer cell.

What Beljanski discovered was that the secondary structure (the hydrogen bonding between the two nucleotides that form the base pairs) can be damaged when something interferes with the hydrogen bond reforming in the replication process.

Beljanski was able to conclude this discovery through a series of tests on the ability of the DNA cell to absorb ultraviolet light (in other words, to make a cell glow like a fluorescent light bulb). He was able to observe that sometimes the hydrogen bonds that have been unzipped for replication to occur do not zip back up. They are prevented from

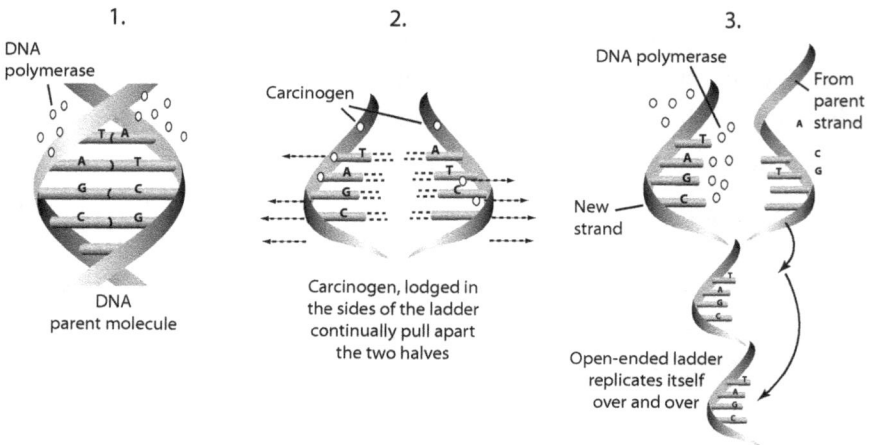

Figure 8: Destabilization

doing so by molecules of chemicals commonly known as carcinogens (cancer causing substances). Carcinogens disallow the hydrogen bonds to be reformed. And therein lies the problem.

Figure 8 shows DNA destabilization:

1. When a DNA parent molecule is closed, it cannot be acted upon by DNA polymerase to create copies of open-stranded DNA. However, once the DNA strand has split itself and the half of the ladder is open, the DNA polymerase that is always there does what it is supposed to do: it causes the open strand to replicate itself. It will continue to do this over and over until the two sides of the DNA ladder can zip themselves back up or until the open side of the ladder is somehow killed or is rendered inert.

2. Since carcinogens are chemicals, they can lodge themselves into the sides of the DNA ladder, and this is why they prevent the hydrogen bonds in the bases, or rungs of the ladder, from reforming: they act as a counter force to the action of the hydrogen bonds. Hydrogen bonds are weak, and the carcinogen residing in the sides of the ladder literally works to pull apart, or torque open, these weak bonds.

3. The hydrogen bonds can't reform, so the open-ended ladder is susceptible to the DNA polymerase which is going to do the job it's supposed to do: make copies of the open-ended rungs of the ladder. So you get an out-of-control copying of the same unzipped DNA molecule.

4. When the DNA in a cell doesn't zip itself back up, a cell's preprogrammed apoptosis somehow gets dismantled.

In other words, the cell doesn't kill itself. It keeps replicating infinitely—the hallmark of a cancer cell.

This is what Dr. Beljanski labeled as "destabilization of DNA," a phenomenon which deals *exclusively* with the secondary structure of the DNA. Its importance cannot be understated. The disruption of the secondary structure of the DNA double helix is a central factor in the creation of cancer. This is revolutionary, and it is a discovery that is "ripe for rediscovery and reappraisal."[15]

In fact, some twenty-five years after Mirko Beljanski first made his observation about the secondary structure and the destabilization of DNA, these phenomena are now being described by many others in the scientific community. [16]

Beljanski's Achievements

This point cannot be stressed strongly enough. Dr. Beljanski made a major discovery when he observed and described destabilization of DNA. First, he observed that when the separation of tightly bound strands of DNA in cellular tissue are contaminated with carcinogens, the result is that the separated strands of the double helix fail to reform in the perfect corkscrew-shaped helix. This failure causes destabilization of the DNA molecule. Second, the destabilized molecule then starts replicating itself over and over with no end, and this causes the cells that contain the destabilized DNA to start replicating themselves over and over with no end. When more carcinogens enter the area, more destabilization of more DNA molecules occur. More cells begin replicating out of control, and eventually a cancerous tumor develops.

As of yet, oncologists do not appear to have adopted Beljanski's cancer-causation finding: that destabilization of DNA is the underlying source of cancer. Consequently, the cause of cancer continues to elude them.

Drs. Watson, Crick, and Wilkins deserved their 1962 Nobel Prize in physiology because they provided all humans with an enormous advancement in understanding the basis of life. Dr. Mirko Beljanski deserved, but never won and can never win, a similar Nobel Prize for tracing the cause of environmental cancer at its core, in the DNA of our cells. Hopefully, history will somehow rectify this mistake.

Case Study: Thyroid Cancer

I met French homemaker, Josiane Chardonnet (Mme. Chardonnet), at the CIRIS picnic, and we discussed the reasons why she had undergone three operations for the removal of thyroid cancer.

Mme. Chardonnet's carcinoma of the thyroid gland kept returning and excisions were required to be performed in 1972, 1975, and 1994. The last operation she underwent removed a giant tumor nine centimeters (cm) (3 ½ inches) in length and seven cm (2¾ inches) in diameter. This last operative procedure brought some bad news with it.

Her cancer surgeon explained that he would perform no more surgeries if Mme. Chardonnet's thyroid tumor returned again. He declared that the interior throat scarring was too great and healing could never take place; thus, any kind of chronic, open ulcer deep in her throat was destined to become infected and that infection definitely would kill her.

There are four types of thyroid malignancies, but Mme. Chardonnet does not know which type she was afflicted with because she never had access to any of the pathology reports relating to her lesions. However, it was made clear by her surgeon and her family physician who practiced internal medicine that she did have thyroid cancer and not a benign thyroid nodule. Because of the size of the third thyroid tumor, Mme. Chardonnet understood that her prognosis was not good.

Josiane Chardonnet affirmed that she needed to carry on an intensive non-toxic, anticancer program in order to prevent a recurrence. Her time was limited. It was then that Mme. Chardonnet heard about Dr. Beljanski's discoveries from both her longtime family physician and the cancer surgeon, both of whom recommended that she take them. The two doctors had suggested these various herbal extracts both for surgical site repair and for purposes of tumor prevention.

Mme. Chardonnet began using three of the herbs immediately after learning about them. Her family physician acquired Beljanski's botanicals for his patient. After speaking with Dr. Beljanski at that time in 1994, the patient's two physicians advised her about the biochemist's recommended quantities of each extract.

Mme. Chardonnet's treatment procedure with herbs was a new strategy in oncology therapy for both of her physicians. Together they made their recommendations as to Mme. Chardonnet's cancer treatment based on what they had heard about remarkable recoveries of patients who had been expected to die very quickly. Anecdotes were circulating about people who were then cancer-free after learning there was no hope of recovery. The two physicians knew very well that Dr. Beljanski was a Ph.D. in biochemistry and not a practicing medical doctor. In 1994, there was still a lack of clinical studies for Beljanski's products, but the surgeon and the internist were willing to risk criticism from their peers in order to help save the life of their patient.

From taking these three products, Mme. Chardonnet has remained happy and well with no sign of thyroid cancer recurrence. When last I checked on her, it was sixteen years since she had that giant tumor removed. She is flourishing. She performs her housework with vigor and continues to take Beljanski's supplements at the same dosage her doctors prescribed. Many patients feel reassured by continuing to take these products, believing that they are reducing the risk of cancer recurrence. Since Dr. Beljanski's products do not have any negative side effects, such practice is safe.

3
The Oncotest:
Beljanski's Cancer Prediction Method

Any good scientist knows that no matter what they uncover at their laboratory bench, from small discoveries to momentous breakthroughs, more questions will follow. Fleming finds penicillin on a petri dish, and the medical community has to then figure out how to use it. Crick, Watson, and Wilkins figure out the double helix of DNA, and that led to over fifty years of massive research into the human genome— the complete set of DNA for the human body, also known as the DNA blueprint.

Dr. Mirko Beljanski was always up for the challenge of "what's next." For Beljanski, once he figured out how DNA destabilization works, the all-important next question became: what if he could take that same mechanism and devise a simple yet very accurate test to identify compounds that could cause and promote destabilization of DNA in a test tube? In other words, what if he could test to see what substances were carcinogenic based on what they did to DNA in a cell?

That would be the ultimate cancer preventative, and the game was on.

The test he developed is called the *Oncotest*. John Hall, Ph.D., writing for the *Townsend Letter for Doctors and Patients* in 2004, reports that the Oncotest, "stands as an elegant, though under-appreciated, development in the history of cancer research."[17] It is a test that can easily and clearly show the carcinogenicity (the ability to cause cancer) of any substance, natural or man-made. It is a very fast test and it is also inexpensive. So why is it ignored?

What is even more remarkable is that Dr. Beljanski made his findings very clear and accessible to the oncological community in his 1983 book, *Regulation of DNA Replication and Transcription*.[18] Unfortunately for the Oncotest, I think it is too accurate, too easy and inexpensive. There are many people who don't want the consuming public to know what is and what isn't truly carcinogenic.

But no matter what any business, corporation, or government wants to hide, the validity of the Oncotest is scientifically proven. As Beljanski's second major scientific discovery, it further helps us understand not only how cancer is created at the cellular level, but also opens the door to a reliable and successful handling of the disease.

The Ames Test for the Screening of Carcinogens

One of the main reasons the Oncotest has been so steadfastly ignored, even in this second decade of the twenty-first century, has to do with the same reason Dr. Beljanski's important multi-breakthroughs in cancer DNA have been largely unrecognized. As Robert A. Weinberg, founder of the Whitehead Institute for Cancer Research and a biology professor at MIT, says in his 1999 book, *One Renegade Cell: How Cancer Begins*, scientists are "now certain" that cancer is caused when genes are damaged through a succession of mutations.[19] We know that isn't correct because destabilization can happen with environmental substances that don't create mutations.

The scientific community has its blind spots, just like anyone does, and it continues to persist in the notion that cancer only comes from mutations. But to privilege mutations means that you are only looking at the *primary* structure of DNA—the sugar-phosphate sides of the ladder held together with a strong covalent bond—not the secondary structure. The secondary structure is the rungs of the ladder made up of the two base pairs—C/G or A/T—held together by the weaker hydrogen bonds and is the part of DNA that is involved in replication. It is in this part that DNA destabilization occurs, and it is in the secondary structure that you can test for carcinogenic substances.

In 1973, the Ames test was developed, and it looked only at the mutations that happen in a certain bacterium.[20] The Ames test was quickly adopted by biochemists and the pharmaceutical industry in that same year and is still widely used by them to this day.

Actually first named the *Salmonella mutagenic test*, it was devised by the then thirty-three-year-old American biologist Bruce Ames, Ph.D. The Ames test is widely applied for screening chemicals occurring in the environment to determine their possible mutagenic activity. While in some cases it reflects carcinogenicity, it was and still is only about 68 percent to 78 percent accurate—and only on carcinogenic substances that promote mutations. Dr. Ames' test determines the effects of a chemical on the rate of mutation in bacterial (Salmonella) microorganisms, which indicate the chemical's likely potential for causing cancer in other living organisms, including humans.

The Ames test works in the following manner: the chemical in question is applied to plates containing growth media for bacteria which lacks the amino acid histidine (a basic amino acid found in many proteins). The growth media on the plates are also inoculated with a special mutant strain of *Salmonella typhimurium*, which requires the amino acid histidine for growth. (The usual wild strain of Salmonella typhimurium is capable of making its own histidine, but this mutant strain is unable to do so.) Cells that mutate back to the wild type, as a consequence of the mutagenic effect of the chemical being tested, are detected by the occurrence of colonies able to synthesize their own histidine and, therefore, able to grow on the media without the amino acid.

Results are obtained in about a week. However, Ames himself realized the limitations of his screening test since it was based only on mutations that occur in these bacteria in the presence of certain chemicals. Ames and others realized that at least 30 percent of known carcinogens are not mutagenic in nature. Some, including Beljanski, knew that nearly 50 percent of carcinogenic substances escape detection by the Ames test.

Dr. Beljanski was skeptical of the Ames test for another reason. He doubted that all mutagenic compounds of various biochemical structures would always induce the exact same type of mutation. This skepticism combined with the fact that so many carcinogenic substances were known not to be mutagenic compelled him to look for a different or complementary explanation.

Carcinogenesis (that which initiates and promotes cancer) is a process Dr. Beljanski was able to initiate in numerous laboratory experiments even when using non-mutagenic compounds. He then compared his lab-produced cells to actual cancer cells removed from living plants, mice, and humans. He found no difference. The idea for the Oncotest was born. Invented around 1976 and described for the first time in a science journal article in 1979, the Oncotest was radically different from all tests existing up to that year.[21]

The Oncotest and Its Advantages

To understand the workings of Dr. Beljanski's Oncotest for identifying carcinogens, we will examine how it functions. Like the Ames test, the Oncotest is an *in vitro* test meaning that it happens in test tubes. It's a method for screening substances for carcinogenic activity based on the hydrogen bonds not reforming in DNA replication.

The idea for the Oncotest came from the wide use of testing of normal cell DNA duplication. This examination method has acquired an often-referenced scientific name: the *Polymerase Chain Reaction,* commonly referred to in biochemistry as the *PCR.* It's what the scientists used as a diagnostic technique in *Jurassic Park* and is used in the popular T.V. series, *CSI.*

When Dr. Beljanski employed the PCR, it was a new tool, but our intrepid researcher quickly figured out another use for it. He used it to compare the different effects of various molecules on purified healthy-cell DNA versus cancer-cell DNA.

But the Oncotest came straight from Beljanski's research on destabilization. As we discussed at length in chapter 2, certain substances keep the replicated DNA strand from reforming back into its stable double-helix formation. When the hydrogen bonds don't reform, they create large gaping loops in the double helix of the DNA strands themselves. These gaping loops create cancerous DNA. And therein lies the simple brilliance of the Oncotest: these large gaping loops allow more light—UV light to be exact—to penetrate the cancerous DNA. It is a well-known phenomenon called *hyperchromicity*. Hyperchromicity is the increase in a molecule's ability to absorb UV light. UV absorption, for example, is increased when the two single DNA strands are being separated. The amount of light penetrating a solution of cancerous DNA mixed with the substance being tested can effectively be measured by a spectrophotometer (a light measuring device).

To make it simple, the more UV light that is absorbed in the DNA, the more carcinogenic is the substance being tested. That is the simplicity of the Oncotest.

Surprising Findings

Once Beljanski was able to observe what happens to DNA in the presence of a carcinogen, he then got busy studying the effects. What he found explains much about why cancerous cells behave the way they do.

DNA that has been isolated and purified from cancer cells always demonstrates a weak but persistent destabilization compared to healthy cells. Such a characteristic explains two particular cancer phenomena observed by microbiologists. The first is that there is an accelerated speed of multiplication in malignant cells.

Have you ever wondered how cancer can sometimes spread so rapidly? It is because the presence of carcinogens *increases* the growth rate of carcinogenic DNA whereas non-carcinogenic substances do not. The Oncotest proved this conclusively.

The process Beljanski discovered is astounding, and it makes perfect sense. As discussed in chapter 2, once the hydrogen bonds between the base pairs of DNA are separated by carcinogens and are unable to zip back up, the enzymes responsible for DNA duplication acquire increased access to the open strands. The enzyme just does what it's programmed to do: make more strands—make more and more DNA copies exactly like the original. In other words, the replication process of a destabilized DNA molecule becomes abnormally accelerated. Worse, the process can be speeded up even more by the presence of *more* known carcinogens. Finally, Beljanski was able to conclude that all documented carcinogens behave in such a manner.

The second phenomenon that Beljanski was able to explain through the Oncotest was that there is an extreme susceptibility of cancerous DNA to carcinogens compared to their healthy counterparts. By contrast, healthy-cell DNA molecules are practically unchanged in their secondary structure, meaning that there is no breakage in the hydrogen bonds. In this case, the double helical strands are not unnaturally separated, and duplication is neither abnormally nor excessively stimulated.

The Oncotest, then, measures two parameters: first, it shows how various substances *affect* or change duplication rates in DNA, and second, it measures those substances which *effect* or bring about a change in the rate of duplication of DNA. Also, Beljanski was able to demonstrate through his test that the destabilization of DNA can occur progressively and with cumulative effects in the presence of mutagenic as well as non-mutagenic molecules.[22] Finally, the Oncotest was able to show that the above-described phenomena are *perfectly reproducible with all DNA from both healthy and cancerous tissues* (whether they be of plant, mammalian, or human origin).[23]

The Danger of Environmental Toxins

The Oncotest was truly a breakthrough invention in the war against cancer. It showed how cancer overwhelms someone when that patient's cellular DNA becomes compromised through destabilization. But that begs the simple question: what, in the end, does *cause* cancer?

A particularly striking result of Beljanski's Oncotest was that many substances which previously were considered to be innocuous (harmless to the human body) were revealed to have carcinogenic potential, depending on their concentrations. At the time of the test's development, Beljanski was quickly able to confirm the carcinogenicity of numerous antibiotics, antimitotics (drugs that inhibit mitosis, or cell division: a common class of chemotherapeutics), hormones, and a large number of environmental substances. I will deal with the environmental hazards first.

Beljanski's opinion was that environmental substances could interfere with hydrogen bonding between the two DNA strands (its secondary structure) and influence the functioning of DNA. Unfortunately, the pollutants and toxic substances which abound in our environment play such a dangerous role. The consequence of so much toxicity is humankind's real and dramatic increase in rates of cancer, autoimmune diseases, toxic metal syndrome, and much more.

All persons living in industrialized and developing countries are exposed to cancer-causing pollutants, commonly called carcinogens. Walking along any street of most major cities around the world, each of us comes into contact with at least a thousand of them. These contaminants promote destabilized DNA.

These toxic substances are found in all aspects of our everyday environment, within our medicines, as well as in a portion of our food and beverages (among other things). Most of them are man-made or are natural substances altered in some way by human intervention. (The exhaust created in a gas-powered combustion engine is an example of the latter.) Additionally and unquestionably we are exposed to cancer-causing radiation through such apparati as full-body scanners at airports, microwave ovens, and cell phones.

There is much more cancer now than there was fifty years ago or even five years ago. Why? The extreme pollution of our modern environment goes hand-in-hand with the considerable increase in serious diseases. Nearly everyone can name classifications of pollutants and even specific carcinogens.

The short list of carcinogens indicated here in **TABLE 2-B** (some are classified as controversial) is merely an example of dangerous substances affecting people, probably on a daily basis:

TABLE 2-B

solar (sun's) radiation	ultraviolet-B and ultraviolet-C light radiation
cosmic rays	chronic electromagnetic field exposure (from cell phones for example)
nuclear radiation	geopathic stress such as magnetic radiation
irradiated foods	dyes found in processed foods
mobile (cellular) telephones	ionizing radiation as from X-rays or microwaves
industrial toxins	fluoridated drinking water or fluoridated toothpaste
pesticide/herbicide residues	blood triglyceride-lowering drug usage

TABLE 2-B *continued*

swimming in polluted water	blood pressure-lowering drug usage
drinking chlorinated tap water	anti-cholesterol drug usage
use of certain antidepressants	artificial sweeteners such as aspartame
immune-suppressive drug usage	prolonged stress which produces harmful chemicals
dietary deficiencies	cigarette smoking
body invasion of parasites	eating smoked or cured foods, e.g. bacon, salami, lox
industrial glues, dyes, solvents, epoxies, thinners, strippers, reducers, and other chemicals	
hormone therapies such as recombinant Bovine Growth Hormone (rBGH) in dairy milk	
mercury (Hg) toxicity from silver dental amalgam fillings or eating Hg-contaminated fish	
indoor air pollution from chemical cleaners as well chemicals in building materials (carpet, plywood, press board or composite board, paint)	
Radiation from X-rays including dental and other health-related X-rays as well as the X-rays your body is now subjected to in airport security.	

Of course, this table is only partial. In fact, there are probably a hundred-thousand more environmental substances that are dangerous but simply remain unknown. They are everywhere: in homes, water, the air, drugs, food, and more. And even if each substance is a weak carcinogen in and of itself and thus not able to induce harm by itself, it is the number of times one is exposed to any carcinogen that can turn a healthy cell into a cancerous one.

Fortunately, we are becoming more aware of the fact that large numbers of man-made chemicals are carcinogenic. The press is now more willing to denounce such carcinogens, and people around the world are already aware of the situation since cancer rates continue to increase and affect more and more people.

Hormones Can Cause Cancer

The second major category of carcinogens are hormones. Enzymatic and hormonal actions play an essential role in the life of the cell. DNA does not initiate cellular operations; it only acts when spurred on by certain enzymes, primary among them DNA polymerase. Hormones, like environmental toxins, exercise influence on DNA duplication. Alone, the DNA is stable, even inert, with a constant structure, troubled just by mutations.

For a long time, scientists have drawn attention to the relationship between an excess of hormones and cancer. In fact, this was noted as early as 1936 by the noted oncologist, Dr. A. Lacassagne, who published his findings in volume 27, page 217 of the *American Journal of Cancer*.

Steroids and other hormones, which give no positive reaction under the Ames test (as they are not mutagenic molecules), all behave as carcinogens when tested with the Oncotest. In fact, steroid hormones strongly stimulate the replication of cancerous DNA isolated from hormonally dependent tissues such as the uterus, adrenal glands, prostate, breast, and ovaries. It should be noted that although it is well-known that hormone treatments are associated with a variety of side effects, Beljanski was among the first to point out that cancer is one of the risks associated with their use. Hormones are necessary, but they must be precisely balanced in the body, and it has now become clear that hormones can increase the incidence of cancer in diverse cases.

To illustrate, women taking synthetic estrogen and progestin as hormone-replacement therapy suffer an increased risk of breast cancer. Furthermore, hormones or similar biological structures (known in biology as analogs) are widely used in the treatment of some cancers where the goal is to interfere with hormones that promote tumor growth.

This underlying risk—that hormone use might promote cancer—is set against their attraction as miracle drugs that can add muscle mass, offset the effects of menopause, delay the aging process, and even play a role in various anticancer therapies.

Of particular interest is the case of steroid hormones (such as testosterone and estrogen in higher doses). They tend to have a carcinogenic effect on cancerous DNA isolated from hormonally dependent tissue (breasts, ovaries, testes, and other organs). They induce both increased ultraviolet absorbance (hyperchromicity) and a strong enhancement of DNA replication and protein synthesis. In contrast, DNA from healthy hormonally dependent tissues and the cancerous DNA from non-hormonally dependent tissues either respond very weakly or not at all to steroid hormones.

The public is subsequently faced with a dilemma when it comes to hormone supplements or hormone replacement therapies; and it is a dilemma of such seriousness that it has gained international attention.[24] Hormones are given to people of all ages for reasons ranging from acne treatment in young people, to contraception, to treatment of hot flashes and menopause in older women. They are in food, meat, milk, butter, eggs, etc. Under the approving eye of the Food and Drug Administration (FDA), hormones fed to cows are a source of cancer.

Recently, some physicians who practice Complementary, Alternative, and Integrative Medicine (CAIM) have emphasized the difference between so-called bio-identical hormones (hormones which have the same structure as those made by the human body) and synthetic or non-bio-identical hormones whose molecular structures differ from those made by the body.

For instance, all birth control pills contain synthetic, patentable hormones, and they are a source of cancer. (Pharmaceutical companies tend to promote and research only non-bio-identical hormones because these types of hormones are patentable, and thus the drug company protects its investment.) Some CAIM physicians believe that synthetic hormones should be avoided in any dosage. But even bio-identical hormones are necessary only in biologically normal doses, and they become dangerous in excessive doses.

Too bad that most conventional physicians tend to prescribe synthetic hormones as a result of promotional pressures in the form of journal advertising, visits from drug company representatives, outright cash gifts, holiday presents, birthday presents, free vacations, massive amounts of drug samples, and so much more largesse. Many physicians are bribable, unfortunately, and the less ethical are not averse to making a lot of extracurricular income from the gifts of pharmaceutical company executives. There is hope on the horizon, however, because the public is becoming informed and starting to protest. This trend of prescribing non-bio-identical hormones is in the process of changing as of this writing. While synthetic hormones may positively affect human health, physicians prescribing them have also caused illness and even death, especially for women.

Two books I recommend that include vital information about bio-identical hormones, authored by the Hollywood actress Suzanne Somers, are *Ageless: The Naked Truth About Bioidentical Hormones*, published in 2006 by Crown Publishers in New York City and *Knockout: Interviews with Doctors Who Are Curing Cancer*, published in 2009 also by Crown.

Pharmaceutical Industry Executives Reject the Oncotest

If the Oncotest is so potent a test for carcinogens, why has Beljanski's cancer prediction method remained obscured?

Unfortunately, industrial interests do not share those same alarms besetting the public about cancer-causing agents. As I have already hinted, the agricultural, chemical, petroleum, and pharmaceutical industries cite the high financial costs to put firm controls in place, along with the complaint that there is the risk of shutting down entire regions of their market activity if the substances they produce are shown to be carcinogenic.

Although the performance of screening tests should be immensely helpful in determining carcinogenic substances in the agrifood and pharmaceutical industry's quality control checks, these tests are not used because they represent a threat to business profits.

Beljanski did offer his Oncotest as an invaluable diagnostic tool to the pharmaceutical industry, only to be rebuffed. The reason executives of major and minor pharmaceutical manufacturers cited for refusing his offer was that the Oncotest "is too sensitive and efficient at detecting the carcinogenic character of any compounds, including drugs." Beljanski's wife, Monique Beljanski, gave me this explanation in the fall of 2005.

The test detects many molecules as potential dangers to people, pets, farm animals, and other organisms, all of which had not previously been recognized, and may continue to be unrecognized. Cynically, one Big Pharma executive higher up in the drug industry told the test inventor: "You're going to put us in jeopardy! Prevention, as far as we're concerned, means keeping quiet." Monique was in a total state of frustration when she described her husband's disappointment at the response.

The Oncotest was also cast off because it presented a direct refutation to the conformist dogma that cancers come only from mutations—which is far from being the general case and, to a large extent, untrue. Furthermore, industrial interests exert a lot of pressure on ruling bodies to maintain the status quo. It is in the financial best interest for the pharmaceutical industry to hold onto maintaining mutagenesis tests to determine carcinogenicity because these ineffective tests make it possible to continue to sell substances that may be carcinogenic but are not mutagenic.[25]

In the face of just such difficulties, Mirko Beljanski was, nevertheless, not one to worry about whether the pharmaceutical industry could profit or not from his new test. Unfazed, he sensed that this breakthrough Oncotest provided an opportunity like none before, and he remained steadfast in his work.

What's Next?

Faster and more sensitive than any other prediction test used to determine carcinogens, the Oncotest offers a vast number of advantages. It highlights potential carcinogenic compounds that fail to be detected by the classical mutagenic tests (such as the Ames Test) which take at least three days to perform and often require several weeks of costly re-examinations on animals in laboratories. Of the two hundred molecules—common items used by consumers almost every day—which were submitted for analysis by the Oncotest, more than thirty-five were found to have carcinogenic potential. Many of them yield positive responses by the Oncotest but are negative by standard mutagenic tests, even though these same substances cause cancer in laboratory animals after three months. (There is also a variant of the Oncotest that can be used to clarify the results of the Ames test available in the notes for those who are interested.[26])

Such an innovative method for screening was radically different from all tests existing at the time, and it proved to be, and still is, both sensitive and rapid. It also became clear that the Oncotest had a very useful application. With it, a researcher could figure out four different possible results of any one substance in terms of how it affects DNA. These are:

1. A substance acts as a carcinogen. The substance, such as nicotine taken into the body directly or indirectly through cigarette smoke, causes an increase in deregulated DNA activity by penetrating and holding open cancerous cellular DNA strands for an excessively long period of time, sometimes even permanently. Destabilization of the DNA of a healthy cell results from long and cumulative exposure to carcinogens (just as it happens in life but not in a fast, *in vitro* test). This carcinogenic effect is exhibited only on DNA that has been destabilized and can become cancerous. It does not take place with normal DNA. That is to say, the duplication of the DNA originating from healthy cells is barely changed, even in the presence of a carcinogen. However cancerous DNA is significantly affected. Subsequently carcinogenic substances selectively target DNA which is already slightly destabilized. All known carcinogens act in this manner in the Oncotest. Other examples include steroid hormones and Vinblastine, a type of cancer drug that stops cells dividing.

2. A substance has a neutral potential. This type of neutral substance has no effect on the duplication of either normal or cancerous DNA. Cholesterol, insulin, and riboflavin are examples of neutral substances.

3. A substance has toxic potential. The adverse substance poisons the polymerase enzyme which performs the DNA duplication. When this kind of toxicity occurs, neither type of DNA (normal or cancerous) is duplicated or replicated. The common herbicides paraquat and diquat are substances with toxic potential.

4. A substance inhibits the duplication of cancerous DNA. There are some substances in nature which inhibit the duplication of cancerous DNA, but at the same time they cause no interference with the healthy DNA's duplication. These would be the ideal anticancer substances, but is there such a substance in nature? That was the "what's next" question that propelled Beljanski into, perhaps, some of the most notable research in his life.

Case Study: Breast Cancer

Breast cancer is the most common malignancy in women, affecting more than one in eight females living in industrialized western nations. Specifically 184,450 American women developed breast cancer in 2008, and approximately 50,000 died from it. (While the case history to follow involves a French patient, we could not learn how many French women had contracted it in that same year.) However, of those fifty-thousand diagnosed but now dead American women, most likely many of them had learned of their health problem much earlier. The disease is most treatable when detected in its earliest stages.

For decades, breast cancer was treated by the Halstead radical mastectomy procedure or a modified radical mastectomy, but the approach during the past three decades has gradually changed to those procedures which are less debilitating. Conventionally, as of this writing, most breast cancer patients are treated with more limited surgery (a lumpectomy which removes the cancer and some surrounding tissue, rather than the entire breast), chemotherapy, and radiation. Women with hormone sensitive breast cancers are usually treated with drugs that reduce the effects of estrogen on the cancer. These include drugs such as tamoxifen or aromatase inhibitors like Arimidex® or Femara®. In addition, more and more women are electing to engage in programs that involve changes in lifestyle, including improved nutrition, exercise, stress management, nutritional supplements, and relatively non-toxic intravenous treatments, such as high-dose, intravenous Vitamin C therapy.

For homemaker Henriette Bouchet (Mme. Bouchet), the myriad of methods for treating breast cancer were of little concern until October 1986, when she discovered a tiny lump in her right breast.

A week later the growth had disappeared, so she paid no more attention to it. But the memory remained.

Mme. Bouchet, like most women, knew that any thickening in any section of the breast could be indicative of malignancy. She counted herself lucky that nothing came from the lump's presence— it just got rid of itself.

Then in February of the following year, a small hollow area or indentation showed up directly in the same area of her right breast. Just under the indentation she found a small growth, the size of a pimple. But the gynecologist who had been attending to her hormonal needs for over twenty-five years refused to acknowledge that any abnormality of the breast was present. "He told me that everything was just fine," explained Mme. Bouchet.

"This gynecologist pacified my fears by prescribing what I now believe was a placebo, for it did nothing for me whatsoever. I was dissatisfied with the treatment for many weeks afterward. I then began to seek more effective care than I had received. Based on follow-up tests that I underwent in June 1987 at an oncological center located in Strasbourg, France, on the Franco-German border, I learned that my situation actually was serious. The medical facility's breast-cancer specialist told me that I had a malignant tumor growing in my right breast. The doctor, a female, said that it was evolving rapidly and had metastasized to lymph nodes in my armpit. She suggested that I required a mastectomy within the next two weeks.

"I was stunned!"

Mme. Bouchet returned home immediately and again contacted her long-standing gynecologist who already knew of her condition since the doctors in Strasbourg had phoned him. "He performed my mastectomy July 2, 1987, and recommended radiation therapy for me to be taken throughout the month of August that year. But I refused it! When next my doctor wanted me to undergo chemotherapy,

I refused that destructive treatment as well. I knew that the chemical poisons of such drug treatment were not for me," she said emphatically.

Having refused radiotherapy and chemotherapy, Mme. Bouchet did not know how to proceed, and for eight months she did nothing except improve every health aspect of her lifestyle that she could: she switched her diet to organic foods, practiced yoga daily, meditated periodically throughout each day, and generally engaged in a holistic way of living. Prior to her surgery, Mme. Bouchet had instructed the surgeon not to remove any lymph nodes, though clinically she appeared to have several lymph nodes involved. She had refused to have them removed because this well-educated woman was aware that the removal of armpit lymph nodes did not improve survival statistics, even though lymph nodes were involved. She was aware that lymph nodes were generally removed by surgeons to help determine the degree of involvement of the cancer, which would help them decide how intensive the rest of their conventional treatment program should be. (For example, they could then answer the question, what chemotherapeutic drugs should be used? How long should they be given?)

Since Mme. Bouchet had determined beforehand that she did not want any conventional treatment other than surgery, this patient decided not to have any of the lymph nodes removed. Such a procedure also spared her possible complications of lymph-node removal, such as chronic swelling of the affected arm, which sometimes occurs in women who have this surgical operation done. Nevertheless, the woman was concerned that cancer cells were still present in her body and she wondered if just the lifestyle changes would be enough to prevent the cancer from growing and spreading.

Eventually returning to her gynecologist, she depended on him to tell her what to do next. The doctor surprised her and did not advise any follow-up surgery but, instead, told Henriette Bouchet to contact Mirko Beljanski to get the herbal products that this microbiologist had discovered. Dr. Beljanski, according to the gynecologist, had published information about a new concept of cancer causation, and certain herbals, alkaloids, or other nutrients he had available would possibly prove useful her. Her physician went on to assure her that he knew of women with breast cancer, ovarian cancer, and other hormonal malignancies who had benefited greatly from taking them.

Conscious of the fact that Dr. Beljanski was a biologist and not a physician, the patient consulted him to evaluate his information and obtain the botanicals he had prepared for counteracting cancer. In mid-1988, Mme. Bouchet decided to avoid receiving any additional conventional cancer treatments including surgery, radiation, or chemotherapy and instead tried Dr. Beljanski's anticancer botanicals. They became a central part of her life and a routine aspect of her nutritional program. She believes that ingesting Beljanski's supplements are as mandatory for her as eating or sleeping. In an emphatic manner, she says, "On July 9, 1988, I took charge of my life."

Since that time, Mme. Bouchet's health has been excellent with no sign of cancer and no evidence of premature aging. She continues to follow various preventive measures against illness, a primary part of which involves the ingestion of no less than three of Dr. Beljanski's products.

4

Beljanski's Breakthrough Botanicals: The Power of the Bolt Molecule for Handling Cancerous DNA

I began this book by addressing the war on cancer. In the preface, I ponder on who is at war with whom. There are many who proclaim that we're winning this war on cancer because we have so many ways to fight the disease. But if that were true, then why are so many people dying, roughly fifteen hundred people a *day* just in the U.S.? [27]

Here we have this disease that, because it seemingly defies a cure but continually takes the lives of so many people, has become a gigantic battleground of money and power. On one side of the battlefield is the pharmaceutical industrial complex with its well-funded and highly influential lobby, Big Pharma. They are accompanied by traditional health professionals who use the usual cancer treatments created by the pharmaceuticals and that we know well: chemotherapy and radiation being prime among them. We healthcare consumers also know that while sometimes drugs and radiation are effective, oftentimes they are not. And these treatments are always accompanied by the awful side effects of which everyone is all too well aware.

On the other side of the field stand the alternative treatments. Again, some are effective but many are not. Some are accompanied by snake-oil hype that touts the "miracle" substance they're peddling is going to cure everything. No one substance on the planet can cure all our ills, and anything that says it can is pure nonsense.

But the fact remains, we're all going to have to face this dreaded disease either in ourselves or in those we love. So is cancer curable? I believe that it is. I also firmly believe that it is going to take the concerted efforts of both sides of this beleaguered and far too bloody battlefield to come up with a treatment that works, consistently and through time.

There is much to overcome. The pharmaceuticals have invested a ton of money into cancer research. That plus those who advertise cures with no scientific backup have made cancer into a "big business" venture because of the massive amounts of money involved in the manufacture and sale of both the natural "cures" and the pharmaceutical drugs.

We are tired of all the hype and the inevitable disappointment. While I side firmly with those alternative natural therapies that are proven to work, we must be careful of all those dishonest practitioners who are out to make a quick buck. We must also educate ourselves on what works, what doesn't, and the failings of the current offerings.

And that is where the genius of Dr. Mirko Beljanski can lead the way.

Outside the Box

In her published article, "The Beljanski Approach: Outside the Box," Monique Beljanski explains one of the great failings of traditional cancer treatments: She states that chemotherapy and radiation are "cytotoxic," meaning they are deadly to almost all fast-dividing cells in our body. The cancer chemicals are worse than toxic since chemotherapy, administered in any concentration—from the lowest to the highest volume and at all potencies—actually stimulates the growth of more cancer.[28] In other words, as Mme. Beljanski explained to me, "At low doses, these treatments happen to destabilize the DNA thereby increasing replication: they behave like carcinogens. At high doses, they act like toxins on the body." To compound the problem, traditional methods of treatment weaken and even destroy the patient's entire immune system at the very moment it is needed most.

There are a number of reasons why chemotherapy often fails on its own merits:

- It burdens the body's detoxification system so that cellular waste products are allowed to accumulate.

- It causes further destabilization of the cancer patient's DNA which allows further out-of-control replication to take place.

- It kills cells by damaging their DNA resistance to other chemicals in addition to the cytotoxic agents.

- It encourages the "tumor suppressor gene" to mutate extraordinarily so that the mutated gene dominates the tumor's growth and disallows any mutated cancer cells from dying. In other words, no apoptosis (cell death) ever takes place. Cancer cells, with the help of the toxic chemicals continue to replicate out of control, thriving inside the victim's tissues and organs.

Dr. Beljanski was well aware of toxic chemotherapy drugs used by oncologists and other medical doctors to treat malignancies. But he also had made it his life's work to find substances that would work hand-in-hand with traditional medicine. He once said, "I want to help people. I want to find harmless ways to do it, but they should work in conjunction with standard therapies." Although Mirko Beljanski was a scientist, not a physician, he had a deep and abiding sense of duty to use science for aiding his fellow human being. His Oncotest, he knew, could have helped prevent cancer by identifying any and all substances that were carcinogenic in nature. But since the industrial and pharmaceutical interests put an effective stop to that, Dr. Beljanski turned his keen and logical mind to another possible use for the Oncotest.

He reasoned that if potentially carcinogenic substances stimulate the replication of cancer DNA cells (the open-looped cells which replicate *ad infinitum*) but not healthy cells, then perhaps the reverse could be true as well. He asked himself the inevitable next question, "What if there were substances able to inhibit the out-of-control replication of the cancerous DNA—that is to say restabilize the cancerous DNA—but not affect the healthy cells?"

Dr. Beljanski turned his attention to finding some substance, some chemical, some botanical, or some other material that would *selectively* take out the cancerous DNA cells without harming the healthy ones. This is exactly what the standard chemotherapy treatments do *not* do. They're not selective but rather equal-opportunity cell destroyers, and that's what makes these treatments so harmful to the human body.

This idea, that there could be a selective cancer-fighting substance, seemed to be an unattainable dream. But therein lies an enormous problem. If you believe that something can't be true, you deny its existence, even if, in fact, the thing you deny is true and real.

What Mirko Beljanski did find, indeed, are two botanicals that he scientifically tested again and again to prove that they do exactly what they purport to do—handle the cancerous, destabilized DNA cells replicating out of control without harming the healthy cells surrounding them. Beljanski's meticulous research opened the door to finding a solution to the problem of traditional cancer treatments lacking selectivity. It is an ideal solution and one that deserves to be examined more closely by both sides of the battlefield.

Introducing the Anticancer Botanicals

During the period when Dr. Beljanski and his wife were concentrating their attention on perfecting the Oncotest, a debate arose among pharmacologists and other doctors around the European continent concerning an African plant, identified botanically as *Rauwolfia vomitoria (R. vomitoria)*. It grew in a vast territory at the mid-sectional belt traversing West Africa, from the Ivory Coast to the Democratic Republic of the Congo. A commercial extract of the herb was rich in reserpine, an alkaloid found in the plant. Alkaloids are any of a class of nitrogen-based organic compounds of plant origin that have pronounced physiological actions on humans. Among them are morphine, quinine, caffeine and strychnine, and these are often used as the basis for medications such as pain relievers and anesthetics. A few of the alkaloids inhibit cell division, such as colchicine, which treats gout, but others of them can also be poisonous, as this short sample list indicates.

A few internists and psychiatrists had been using reserpine to treat patients with high blood pressure and psychiatric disorders. At that time, questions arose among the involved therapists as to whether the reserpine component was carcinogenic, and that question sparked a hot debate in the medical community. Nobody knew, but many scientists conjectured, about the alkaloid's toxicity as a carcinogen.

Dr. Beljanski was intrigued by the debate about the reserpine alkaloid as well. In order to form his own opinion, he decided to evaluate the plant's characteristics through the use of his Oncotest. With this test, the husband and wife team definitely had a leg up on their fellow scientists in regard to finding out quickly if that particular reserpine alkaloid was harmful or not. Their first task was to acquire a small quantity of this plant extract, which they were able to do within a week.

Upon carrying out a biochemical analysis of a commercially available reserpine-containing extract of *R. vomitoria*, Mirko and his team observed something odd. All living substances react to DNA at a certain rate. Scientists have discovered that this reaction rate shows up as a curve called "the kinetics of the curve," when DNA is synthesized. The *R. vomitoria* curve looked abnormal, so Beljanski asked himself why. One possibility for the abnormality in the graph was an intrusion of plant growth impurities, contaminants in the soil, or a mixture of compounds. So Mirko suggested to Monique that they purify the extract, separate the various elements in the plants, called fractions, and then test each fraction separately using his Oncotest. These procedures took considerable time and energy, but the low cost and excellent efficiency of the Oncotest made their little intellectual game worthwhile. In the end, they reasoned that the extract contained a mixture of substances called alkaloids that had conflicting effects.

In reviewing the results of these experiments, Mirko and Monique were surprised to find that not only did one fraction of the extract, labeled *1-A*, exhibit carcinogenic potential, but a second fraction, marked *2-A*, whose nature they had not yet established, *completely prevented* cancerous DNA synthesis. Eventually, Beljanski was able to identify marker *2-A* as the alkaloid Alstonine, and it did something they had postulated but had never found before—it inhibited the replication cycle of the destabilized cell. Even more astounding, the alkaloid was indifferent to healthy cells. It only acted on cells that were cancerous or about to become cancerous.

Without DNA replication, a cell whether normal or cancerous, cannot multiply. So the team predicted that because it inhibited replication of a bad cell, the *2-A* fraction might suppress malignant tumors. This turned out to be the case. Beljanski found that the Alstonine molecule stopped cultures of cancer cells from growing *in vitro*—in fact, the cell cultures of cancer shrunk and disappeared.

Monique succinctly put it to me again when I met with her in the summer of 2006. It had been about three decades since those experiments, but her excitement was still palpable. She said, "That second *Rauwolfia vomitoria* fraction of *2-A* beautifully illustrated what a cancer-fighting substance should be!"

At the beginning of their investigations, the Beljanskis and their research team studied several alkaloids from the same botanical family, or closely related to the first one. But for various laboratory reasons, they finally concentrated on the *Rauwolfia* plant extract itself.

Finding the "Bolt" Molecule

At first incredulous about these results, Mirko and his team checked their experimental procedures repeatedly and under various conditions. The results came up with the same, selective effects each time, and they decided that they had discovered something significant.

The researchers then carried out further analytical procedures to establish the molecular characteristics of each constituent in *Rauwolfia vomitoria*. This process was effective in isolating the important component that would later be called a "bolt molecule." They then determined the chemical structure of the plant's specific active factor—again it was Alstonine—which selectively inhibited the growth of cancerous DNA. Then because part of the *R. Vomitoria* is toxic, they developed the painstaking process to produce a highly purified extract that removes any harmful residue.

Bolt molecules, as defined by Dr. Beljanski, are the actual individual chemical constituents in a formula which bring about healing of malfunctioning cells, tissues, organs, and/or whole body parts.

After months of painstaking work, the researchers fully realized that finding the plant's active factor may be of great therapeutic importance to victims of cancer. They labored diligently to acquire a much greater quantity of the plant and to purify larger amounts of the active component. Ten years of hard work led to numerous additional analyses and tests as well as toxicology studies. The results were consistent and always striking: the concentrated and highly purified *Rauwolfia vomitoria* extract is rich in selective bolt molecules that inhibit almost all types of cancer cells. It also has a preference for hormonal tissues.

The Second Anticancer Alkaloid

Once Dr. Beljanski had discovered the bolt molecule in *R. vomitoria*, he went looking for other botanicals with the same types of alkaloids. He found a second promising substance that was derived from the powdered bark of a Brazilian rainforest tree. The plant is named Pao pereira (*Geissospermum velosii*), and knowledge about it has become invaluable for cancer treatment. Through another long series of laboratory tests, Beljanski and his team found that the bark of the Pao pereira, extracted and purified, induced apoptosis with its "bolt" molecule, Flavopereirine. [30] This is invaluable when fighting cancer because the most effective way to stop a cancer cell from replicating itself indefi-nitely is to get it to kill itself!

Because of their consistently promising results, Dr. Beljanski decided to focus his full attention on studying these two alkaloid extracts in depth. They have many properties in common, not the least of which is their ability to be selective and remain non-toxic while combating cancerous cells. The science of how they work is of course very complex, and one of the most important differences between the two substances is that the smaller Pao molecule is able to cross the human blood-brain barrier, while the *R. vomitoria* alkaloid cannot. (The blood-brain barrier is a tight cellular seal that prevents foreign chemicals from easily getting into the brain. Poisons cannot reach the brain because of it.)

This is important to know when dealing with brain cancers because the small Pao molecule provides help in such cases but *Rauwolfia* does not. More important, however, is that the two alkaloids have a wonderfully synergistic effect when put together, the one inhibiting the replication cycle, the other inducing cell death. It's a one-two punch against the cancer cell that Beljanski found to work over and over in his laboratory experiments.

Demand Grows

Once physicians and patients found out about them, they clamored to obtain the two botanicals. In his book, *Extraordinary Healing*, Stephen Coles, M.D., reports that the first "bolt" molecules were discov-ered around the mid-1980s. The first requests from desperate patients looking for something to save their lives came to Dr. and Mme. Beljanski around 1986, and for almost a decade, they dispensed their botanical extracts throughout Western Europe, entirely as the result of word of mouth. Beljanski never did anything other than what a scientist should do—write up his findings in peer-reviewed scientific or medical journals. Dr. Coles makes it clear that Beljanski never publicized his findings or advertised the botanical extracts, but doctors reading about them in the scientific journals would contact him, asking him to supply them with his formulas. People would hear about the curative effects of the botanicals and contact the Beljanski laboratory, begging this microbiologist for his nutritional supplements.[31]

For over thirty years, the two botanicals, Pao pereira and *Rauwolfia vomitoria,* have successfully been used to manage cancer and viral pathologies throughout Europe. They are well-known by doctors and patients on that continent, yet Dr. Beljanski's products still remain relatively unknown in the United States because of overwhelming monopolistic practices of America's version of Big Pharma. The pharmaceutical industry has a vested interest in keeping Beljanski's findings out of mainstream literature on cancer. But doctors in the U.S., like their counterparts in Europe twenty years ago, are starting to increasingly read more about the success of Beljanski's discoveries and are wanting additional information.

After witnessing the satisfaction of European patients during my visit to France in September 2003 and more recently during May 2011, I vowed to vigorously but strictly voluntarily devote my time and efforts to raising awareness of the American public to the remarkably turbulent history, yet magnificent oncological and virological success, of this pair of herbal breakthroughs. These alkaloid extracts have already saved so many people in Europe from dying of malignant tumors, I have made it my mission to help the American medical consumer become aware of the possibilities they offer. I have never received any financial remuneration from the Beljanski Foundation or from Dr. Mirko Beljanski's relatives, except when we interviewed together at a restaurant and Sylvie or Monique Beljanski paid the restaurant tab. I use these herbs myself as an anticancer preventive, and I pay for Beljanski's supplements the same as does any other consumer or health professional.

Understanding the Bolt Molecules

In order to understand how these anticancer "bolt" molecules selectively penetrate the pathological cell and not the normal cell, it is important to know that when a cell is in the process of becoming cancerous, several meaningful changes occur. Such abnormal alterations are significant because they characterize malignancy. These changes are as follows:

a. the membrane's porosity alters from non-porous in healthy cells to porous in cancer cells.

b. the cytoplasmic pH* and Rh* are reversed. The cytoplasm is the thick liquid that holds all the various elements of a cell, called organelles.

c. the cell nucleus enlarges into an unusual size. Because the cell's DNA becomes destabilized, large scale, out-of-control replication starts taking place.

A healthy, non-porous cell will *not* be penetrated by the bolt molecules. A cancerous cell is porous, so it is able to be penetrated by all sorts of molecules, good and bad. That's why carcinogens in the presence of a destabilized cell are so detrimental and, conversely, when the bolt molecules present themselves at the cellular wall of a cancer cell, the cancer cell will allow it to enter as it allows any other molecule to enter.

But the bolt molecule has a different effect on the DNA of the cell than a carcinogen. The carcinogen, as we saw in chapter 2, disallows the weak hydrogen bonds of the DNA cell to close up after they have replicated themselves (the destabilization effect). The open strand of DNA will replicate over and over again out of control. In one study,

---

* pH - potential of Hydrogen. H is a measure of the activity of hydrogen ions (H+) in a solution and, therefore, its acidity or alkalinity. The pH value is a number without units, between 0 and 14, that indicates whether a solution is acidic (with a pH less than 7) or alkaline (with a pH more than 7)

* Rh – Symbol expressing the oxidoreduction potential within a body, such as a cell; it relates to flow of electrons and is different in normal cells and cancer cells

for example, Beljanski found that the "unwinding of the cancer DNA is perfectly proportional to the increase in DNA synthesis." [32] As noted in chapter 3, the more DNA unwinds, or unzips, the more DNA replication and reformation (otherwise known as DNA synthesis) occurs. That is why cancer cells replicate far faster than healthy cells—the cancer cells have DNA whose strands are constantly unwound, thus the increase in cell production.

The bolt molecules work together to kill the out-of-control cells, with the highly positive effect of *eliminating multibillions of cancer cells.* As I said at the beginning of this chapter, I believe that cancer can be cured.

There were numerous studies done by Beljanski's team to show the effectiveness of the bolt molecules. Beljanski showed how each alkaloid attaches exclusively to tumors in both plants and mice. For example, his team was able to obtain photographs which are marvelously illustrative of the fact that healthy brain cells (specifically astrocytes) are *not* penetrated by the alkaloid, while cancerous cells (in this instance, components of a glioblastoma brain tumor) are quickly penetrated. The penetrating alkaloid enters through the membrane surrounding the nucleus of the cancer cell and destroys the entire cell that provides housing for the cancer. This phenomenon is even more visible under ultraviolet light. The cancer-targeting alkaloids share the property of being naturally fluorescent (under UV light, they glow like a fluorescent light bulb) and Beljanski was able to photograph the phenomenon.

In Vitro Studies Among Cancer Cells and Normally Healthy Cells

There is a certain protocol that scientists employ when studying a substance that will potentially be used for human consumption. It is first tested *in vitro*, meaning cells that are to be studied are isolated in some special tubes, and experiments on such cells are conducted. When the *in vitro* tests show promise, then the researcher turns to study the substance *in vivo*, literally in living things. *In vivo* happens most often in laboratory mice but will occur in other living organisms as well. Once the substance proves to be effective *in vivo*, then the substance moves to human trials, where it is tested on humans afflicted with the disease being studied.

For *in vitro* tests, microbiological researchers most often use healthy and cancerous human cells able to be cultured in laboratories. This makes it possible to conduct numerous very useful experiments in order to understand the factors related to certain items. Such items include, for example, how the tested products work, the correct dosages, their eventual toxicity, and a great deal more. All types of cells are thus available and such a controlled study is largely conducted in laboratories where conditions are most ideal for achieving accurate results.[33]

After Beljanski found that the Pao pereira and *Rauwolfia vomitoria* herbal extracts reduced UV absorption and replication activity in cancer DNA using the Oncotest, he then proceeded to test the two extracts in a fairly extensive series of *in vitro* tests. Over and over the research proved the same thing: *growth inhibition takes place in cancer cells by coming in contact with the two Beljanski-discovered alkaloids while healthy cells remain untouched.*[34]

Numerous *in vivo* experiments showed Beljanski's team that the two alkaloid extracts did not attach to normal DNA, and more importantly, did not show any signs of toxicity. In a study done late in Beljanski's life on the Pao pereira extract, and whose results were published posthumously in 2000, the extract, which the microbiologist dubbed "the plant-derived anticancer agent PB-100," showed inhibited cell growth in sixteen distinct cancer cells anywhere from 83.78 percent in the designated "ZR-75-1" breast cancer cell to 99.64 percent inhibition in the "U251" brain cancer cell.

From colon cancer to liver, kidney, skin, ovary, pancreas, prostate and thyroid cancers, Pao Pereira showed remarkably high *in vitro* kill rates for all these cancer cells—all in the upper 80 percent to the mid

90 percent range. And according to Stephen Coles, different laboratories in the years following that 2000 study have conducted several similar experiments with the Pao extract. These subsequent studies not only confirmed the high percentage of cancer cells dying but in keeping with the selective properties of the botanical, under the same *in vitro* conditions, normal cell lines were not destroyed. [35]

Time and again, the *in vivo* studies clearly showed that human clinical trials are justified.

In Vivo Studies Among Plants

During the late 1970s and early 1980s—perhaps over a six-year period—a crucial series of mental attitudes developed for the Beljanski research group. The group's members strongly sensed and discussed that they were onto a piece of anticancer science that was both fundamental and vital for the health and welfare of all humankind. For Mirko and Monique Beljanski as team leaders, it was the restarting of an intellectual adventure, delving deeply into life's great unknown.

In 1978, the Beljanski's were unceremoniously removed from the Pasteur Institute. While that was a secure situation in terms of finance, the animosity between Beljanski and Monod made it impossible for Beljanski to continue his work at the famed institute. With faith and enthusiasm, the scientist and his wife found a new home. Their first ten years of independence was with an independent research facility at the University of Châtenay-Malabry School of Pharmacy outside of Paris. Then, they spent another ten years in an independent, private laboratory in St. Prim, a small village south of Lyons that was created by CIRIS. Over the next twenty years, the husband and wife team along with their coworkers became excited with new findings coming to them almost daily. Their enthusiasm became infectious, especially among their five newly hired fellow investigators engaged in studies involving plant cancers.

A woman who had worked next door in the plant oncology laboratory of the Pasteur Institute, the studious researcher Liliane Le Goff, Ph.D., joined in the Beljanski group's enthusiasm. Although she knew that Jacques Monod opposed Dr. Beljanski's concepts. Dr. Le Goff found the courage and perseverance to dedicate twenty-six years of her life collaborating with Beljanski. She ended up spending more time in Mirko's small laboratory than in her own at the Pasteur! Working with Beljanski was a source of intellectual happiness for her.

Furthermore, Dr. Le Goff soon persuaded another researcher from the Jussieu University's Faculty of Science to participate with the Beljanski group as well. Because of the valuable information she observed being uncovered, Madame Y. Aaron-Da-Cunha, Ph.D., also became attached and devoted to Beljanski and his team. She turned into a team member and worked diligently despite the external pressure that was exerted on her by the Pasteur Institute's director to end her collaboration. All three researchers, Dr. Le Goff, Dr. Y. Aaron-Da-Cunha, and Dr. Mirko Beljanski, co-authored and published many biochemistry papers relating to plant cancer induction and plant cancer inhibition.[36]

Plant cancers are induced by a soil-derived type of bacteria known as *Agrobacterium tumefaciens (A. tumefaciens)*. Here is what happens: A wound to the stem or the root of a plant incites an influx of plant hormones which destabilize the plant's DNA.[37] This wound excites the *A. tumefaciens* bacteria to inject a type of RNA that tends to become oncogenic, in other words, it causes tumors to develop. When the bacteria inject the oncogenic RNA into the plant, a tumor begins to form shortly thereafter.[38]

The research team found, not surprisingly, that both the Pao and *Rauwolfia* bolt chemical extracts are 90 percent successful at inhibiting these botanical tumors, all without negative or toxic effects on the plant, which continues normal, healthy development.

The four main research teammates consisting of the two Beljanskis, Dr. Le Goff, and Dr. Aaron-Da-Cunha also demonstrated the important role of plant hormones in the process of introducing and inhibiting cancer in plants. Plant hormones may neutralize the anticancer effect of the Beljanski extracts, depending on the amount of each product put into play by the investigators, a fact that was proven to be true later in human hormonal tissue as well.

Many experiments were conducted over the years by the Beljanski research team to better understand the mechanisms and diverse interactions that come into action during this process. It was concluded that the *Rauwolfia* extract could be as valuable for healing cancer in horticulture as it is for sustaining the health of mammals and man.

Massive amounts of botanical research were carried forward and, indeed, it would behoove the world of agriculture to continue the research Beljanski began to find natural, non-toxic ways to treat the scourge of cancer in plants.

In Vivo Anticancer Studies in Mice

When the original members of Beljanski's team left the Pasteur Institute in 1978 and went to work for ten years at the pharmaceutical university, they were able to obtain live laboratory animals, making it possible to study cancer in experimental specimens. While they received no funding from the university or the CNRS (the National Center for Scientific Research, the organization that funds research at the Pasteur Institute as well as other scientific organizations in France), they obtained a contract with the French army to investigate ways of protecting against radiation poisoning—the results of which you will learn about in the next few chapters. This move to the Malabry School of Pharmacy proved to be important because it became possible to buy hundreds of laboratory-raised mice and conduct many different types of experiments on them involving the transplantation of various types of cancer cell lines.

With laboratory mice at Beljanski's disposal, and because the *Rauwolfia vomitoria* and Pao pereira extracts' anticancer effects were demonstrated *in vitro*, the research team set out to investigate anticancer activity *in vivo*. Following well-established conventional experimental protocols, the research team grafted dozens of different types of cancers into the mice, including lymphoma, malignant breast tumors, and others. The guideline used for determining how well these *in vitro* treatments work was comparing the percentage of mice that survived in excellent condition at the end of the three-month trial period to a control group that had not received any treatment.

Depending on the doses of *Rauwolfia vomitoria* and Pao pereira extracts used as therapy, the tumor-ridden mice showed high survival rates in a wide variety of different cancers. In one study, cell lines from a type of lymphoma were transplanted into mice. The mice were given the *R. vomitoria* extract, and at the "highest doses, up to 80 percent of the mice treated [with the compound] survived for ninety days, whereas all of the untreated mice were dead by day forty....All mice that did not survive had developed tumors...Cured mice survived in excellent condition." No secondary toxic effects appeared. The herbal extracts prolonged the lives of numerous mice and saved the lives of many others, all of which had been victimized in their cages by transplanted cancers. The affected mice also exhibited no side effects, no nausea, no hair loss, no cracks in the mucous membranes, nothing at all destructive to the quality of life.

Columbia University Studies on Prostate Cancer

Dr. Mirko Beljanski passed away in October of 1998, and I will relate the story of his death in a later chapter. But I believe it is important that additional studies that have been done on his anticancer molecules be reported on in this current chapter to give you the full scope of the work being carried out in such prestigious American institutions as Columbia University's Center for Holistic Urology and the Cancer Treatment Centers of America. I do so to honor the late Dr. Mirko Beljanski and also to suggest to those researchers reading this material that there is much work to be done to first recreate the Beljanski team's experiments and then take such data into further research on the healing properties of these two alkaloid extracts.

Aaron Katz, M.D., director of the Center for Holistic Urology, was introduced to Beljanski's approach through the same well-respected physician that introduced them to me: Michael B. Schachter, M.D., of Suffern, New York. Dr. Katz became interested in Beljanski's products after meeting with Dr. Beljanski's widow, Monique, and his daughter, Sylvie. He told the two women that his patients had continually badgered him with questions about various products, and he had embarked on empirical research to discover what worked and what didn't. Dr. Katz reports that Sylvie Beljanski gave him a number of her father's peer-reviewed scientific articles with his research results, which interested him greatly. He told Sylvie that in order for Beljanski's work to be accepted by American doctors, all the painstaking research would have to be repeated. [40]

The Columbia University team got to work, and they were not disappointed. The first results were published in the November 2006 issue of the *International Journal of Oncology*. Titled "Antiprostate Cancer Activity of a Beta-Carboline Alkaloid Enriched Extract from *Rauwolfia vomitoria*," the article reported that in both *in vitro* and *in vivo* studies of the *R. vomitoria* extract on the human prostate cancer cell line (technically called LNCaP), tumor volumes were decreased by 58 to 70 percent, depending on the dose of *R. vomitoria* administered to the mice. The extract was showing the same kind of results that Beljanski's research had shown twenty years earlier.

Columbia's research team then tested the Pao pereira extract both *in vivo* and *in vitro* and, again, formed the same conclusion as Beljanski. The Pao pereira extract, enriched with the active alkaloid Flavopereirine, "significantly suppressed cell growth and induced apoptosis (cell death) in LNCaP cell cultures as well as in LNCaP tumor xenografts (the transplanting of living cells, tissues, or organs from one species to another)."[41]

The results were again published in the 2009 issue of the *Journal of the Society of Integrative Oncology* that reported the same findings: both the *R. vomitoria* and the Pao pereira extracts Beljanski and his team developed showed "significant anticancer activity in certain preclinical models," enough to justify a human trial for men suffering from prostate cancer.[42] The preliminary human trial was completed by Dr. Aaron Katz, M.D., director of the Columbia Center for Holistic Urology sometime in 2009, and the results were written up by Melissa Burchill, Rd, CDN, in *Integrative Medicine*. Ms. Burchill reports that Dr. Katz noted that "We now know that [the two extracts, combined], significantly lowered PSAs (the markers that may indicate prostate cancer) in a twelve-month period."[43]

There is also an interesting piece of information in the 2009 *Integrative Oncology* article that reported on the trial then in progress that I would be remiss in not reporting. According to that article, "the tumor-suppressing effect of the Pao pereira extract was apparently lost at the highest dose (50 mg/kg/d)..."[44] While I do not know how that particular dosage in the *in vivo* trials in mice translates to human dosages, it is important to note that the reader is advised to take any treatment under the care of a knowledgeable and caring physician, either traditional or alternative, who can monitor the dosages.

Dosage issues aside, the Columbia studies lend a great deal of scientific credence to the work the Beljanski team performed in France. These studies help us all to better understand the science behind the excellent effect these purified extracts can provide anyone diagnosed with cancer or who show early warning signs, also called markers, for cancer.

Whatever must be done to understand, recreate, and apply Beljanski's research, it is imperative that we demand it be done. These anticancer results were possible because of the selectivity of Beljanski's "bolt" molecules for cancer cells alone. He found them to be even more effective when combined with conventional cancer treatments—a subject I will take up in-depth in the next chapter.

French Doctors Prescribe the Botanicals

Dr. Beljanski was aware of his good fortune in uncovering the two alkaloids containing "bolt" molecules, the ideal substances to fight cancer because they only target cancer cells and thus do not have side effects associated with them. From the time that reports began to emerge about the success of some cancer patients with Beljanski's botanicals, doctors from every corner of France (some of them en-lightened oncologists) solicited the Beljanski team members, to get help for themselves, their families, and their patients, including other nature-derived supplements Beljanski had developed.

Unfortunately, the popularity of his discoveries was dangerous both for the Beljanski team members and for the individual medical doctors who tried to help patients with Dr. Beljanski's supplements. France, even more so than in the U.S., opposes the practice of holistic medicine or even discussions of any therapies using CAIM (Complementary, Alternative, and Integrative Medicine). Politicians in France are closely associated with that country's pharmaceutical industry lobbyists with their big money bribes even more so than in the United States. As with American politicians, the French politicians take very large sums of drug industry lobbyists' funds. These lobbyists make sure to use their money, power, and persuasion to get European bureaucrats to go so far as to take away a physician's license to practice medicine when that practice fails to prescribe or dispense copious quantities of drug products.

This untenable situation was created under the Vichy government during World War II. Named "the Order of Doctors" (*l'Ordre de Medecins*), it carries out a witch hunt of sorts on French medical doctors who practice medicine employing a holistic approach. They do so by monitoring what is prescribed. In contrast to common medical pro-cedure in many states in the U.S., doctors in France do not have the right to sell products from their offices or to even give them as gifts to their patients. Samples of drugs to physicians are fewer too. The pharmaceutical industry, directly or indirectly, finances most public officials. Their interests conflict with those of the patient. From this perspective, the political position of doctors in France is quite fragile.

Despite all of these adverse conditions involving restrictions on freedom and civil rights, about 450 medical doctors were sufficiently impressed with Beljanski's results, along with what they observed in patients, that they risked their careers to recommend them in order to help their patients. In discussions among themselves, these holistic-thinking French medical doctors agreed to run the risk of making some serious enemies in their professional organization. It is thanks to such brave physicians that at least twenty thousand sick French people were able to receive their self-administered herbal treatments.

More than bravery, however, the real story behind these anticancer botanicals is the passion that Mirko Beljanski had for his biological research.

Mirko the Man, a Passionate Researcher

I have shown throughout this book that Dr. Beljanski was an indefatigable experimenter in his scientific endeavors. He constantly verified his results, varying experimental conditions along every conceivable parameter, and endlessly starting over. He knew, more so than any of his colleagues, there was no room for error.

In the book *Chronique d'une Fatwa Scientifique*, Beljanski's wife and staunch assistant states the following:

> *His whole life, Mirko said and showed that one can and one must do something, must fight, to find a solution. When he would later go up against diseases considered to be incurable, his energy, never lacking, would effectively find a solution. His can-do spirit would break down the barriers of habit, convention, ease, and*

fatalism. He left nothing to chance. He wanted to anticipate and to control. He always maintained a vision of the future which he projected onto the present moment. Behind each isolated fact, he saw all of its possibilities [...] In matters of science Mirko could never rest as long as there was something to be done.

Often, his best qualities would work against him: he would annoy, bother, he would take logic to an extreme and would suffer the consequences. Many years later, he would take science to a higher level, requiring that it serve man so as to diminish suffering, disease, and medical costs. [45]

Better than anyone, Mirko Beljanski knew that, like an artist, the researcher is an adventurer. He must break with old customs, ways of thinking, and inherited ideas. Every person, thing, idea, and fact must be viewed with a fresh eye through a personal lens, separate from the norm. Each judgment—beginning with his own—must be endlessly questioned. The scientist like the artist journeys to new horizons, but it is a lonely road. As their estimations of value are unique, so too, are their criticisms. Solitude is the price of such individualism: it maintains and facilitates doubt, continual questioning, and the search for truth.

To create, one must be uncomfortable, anxious, and driven by an internal imperative. Instead of seeking constant comfort in what is known, a person of vision uses acquired knowledge only as a spring board. The known must also be surpassed and conclusions constantly reevaluated in order to venture into the search for a new form of thought or expression. This almost always requires putting oneself in direct conflict with others, renouncing the assurance of friendships easily born of the shared ideas in vogue. Breaking new ground is almost masochistic in nature, and is an act which very few tolerate and which is not suffered well by those in one's immediate entourage. A break in one's thinking quickly leads to a break in certain ties that normally bind men and women together.

Certainly, marginalization occurs when one thinks or works differently than the status quo. But for those who take risks and live life on their own terms, there is no other choice.

Dr. Mirko Beljanski kept himself walled off from pressures, impervious even to threats from the scientific community when he made discoveries that ran contrary to established dogma or conventional wisdom. His fortitude and tenacity will be forever appreciated by all those who avail themselves of his discoveries.

The Uncurable Myth

It is true in science, as in art, that they are laden with conformists who use their talent to make for themselves a socially comfortable situation. These types of people are the biggest enemies of innovation, and there is an army of them. It is they who populate those on the side of the war who claim the only effective treatments for cancer are toxic, and that cancer, ultimately, isn't curable. For them, to cure cancer means the loss of billions of dollars.

And that is, at heart, what keeps the "war on cancer" firmly entrenched. Money. The producer of the most-read Internet health newsletter in the United States, Joseph Mercola, D.O., states: "They [the drug makers] want you to feel frightened for your health, as that is a very powerful motivating emotion. The goal of the campaign [drug advertising] is to create a picture where relying on them [again, the drug makers] for the solution (to the health issue they made you fearful of) is necessary. This creates a dependency and annuity that enriches their bottom line." [46]

A similar sentiment is shared by Samuel Epstein, M.D., in his 1998 book, *The Politics of Cancer Revisited*. In the book's dynamic introduction he makes the assertion that: "the National Cancer Institute and the American Cancer Society have misled and confused the public and Congress by repeated false claims that we are winning the war against cancer, and these are claims made to create public and Congressional support for massive increases in budgetary appropriations."

Dr. Epstein is mindful of the destruction brought to all peoples by an inability of the medical profession to practice out of their restrictive box which confines them to conventional treatment strictly using chemotherapies, radiation, and other unnatural/poisonous agents. With great sadness, Samuel Epstein, M.D., concludes:

> Cancer is a major cause of misery and death. Moreover, the distribution of hardship falls unevenly on those with least resources. Cancer cannot be explained away as something that just "happens" to people. Rather, we need to see many cancers as being caused by exposure to carcinogens in the workplace, in consumer products, and in the general environment. These cancers are largely preventable—if the real nature of their causes is understood and the fight against them becomes a political priority. [47]

To say that cancer is uncurable is a myth perpetrated by scheming, greedy people who want to keep the cancer machine alive. That is evil at its core.

But evil will always crumble in the light of truth. I believe now, without doubt, that the research done by Dr. Mirko Beljanski and his dedicated team of researchers has given us not only a way to treat cancer but to *prevent* the disease from occurring in the first place. We now know the power Beljanski's natural supplements provide. Mirko Beljanski went a step further and proved that true integrative therapies, applying both his botanical formulas to the traditional treatments we have used for over sixty years, could have astounding effects.

But it will take all of us to step aside from the prevailing beliefs that we hold about cancer, look directly at the data available to us now, and demand that more studies be done to finish the work of Dr. Beljanski. Let's find a way to combat this deadly disease so that it becomes not the frightening monster that we perceive, but the very treatable and ultimately curable disease that it truly is.

With Beljanski's natural and non-toxic supplements leading the way, we need to fight to bring to the forefront cancer therapies that are proving themselves scientifically to be more effective for treating cancer than conventional oncological treatments. We need anticancer remedies that improve the quality of patients' lives rather than force them to suffer the ill effects of surgery, radiation, and poisonous chemicals.[48] In other countries there are traditional, alternative, and complementary medical doctors working together to extend the cancer patient's life, to keep him or her vital and active, and most predominantly to effectively render treatment without adverse side effects. We in the United States need to adopt these viewpoints and ways of working together if we want to win *our* battle against cancer.

The means are available.

Case Study: Prostate Cancer

For eleven years, Henri Boiteux, Ph.D., a resident of southern France and currently retired as Professor of Physics at the University of Paris, had been Director of Research at the CNRS, and for eleven years the Administrator of a prominent Cancer Treatment Center of Villejuif near Paris. The CNRS in France is equivalent to the National Institutes of Health (NIH) in the United States. As administrator of the Center, invariably Dr. Boiteux had participated in executive decisions about the awarding of research grants for evaluations of medical therapies. He studied all aspects of treatment for most types of diseases, including cancer. Dr. Boiteux received exposure to every means of health care available worldwide. If he personally had need of some sort of therapeutic intervention for illness, Dr. Boiteux certainly was free to choose the method he believed to be most beneficial for his own healing.

This university professor, so very knowledgeable about medical treatment and other life-saving issues, preserved his own life by electing to use the natural products developed by Dr. Mirko Beljanski. Professor Boiteux assured that, for himself, nothing else would do. He said, "My experience at the CNRS—which brought me in close contact for more than a decade with the most progressive therapies—taught me the best, the mediocre, and the worst treatments. I want what works!"

The Personal Case History Provided by Henri Boiteux, Ph.D.

In June 1994, the professor was told by an urologist local to the area of his country village that at age seventy-three, he was affected by prostate cancer.

"My doctor, a conventionally-practicing country physician who specialized in the human urogenital system, said to me, 'The only treatment you can receive for your malignant prostate gland is radiotherapy. Your cancer is five years advanced, and because of the tumor's particular location, it is inoperable.'

"I did not doubt the accuracy of the doctor's diagnosis nor the possible efficacy of the treatment he was offering," Professor Boiteux assured me. "But radiation was not a treatment in which I had any confidence. It would have been the treatment of last resort for my prostate. I knew of other men who had failed to benefit from receiving it, and I knew from my eleven years at the Cancer Treatment Center of Villejuif that a treatment from radiotherapy was rarely permanent and likely inadequate."

Since his patient's prostate tumor was estimated to be present for so many years, the professor's urologist admitted to being dubious about administering radiation right away and decided to wait. "Instead," Professor Boiteux said, "my doctor added a further recommendation which was: 'You require some further investigatory work because I want to learn if any metastases of the cancer has occurred over this long interval of non-treatment.'

"Consequently, the urology specialist had me go through a lot more testing at the local hospital and at various medical laboratory offices some distances from my home," says the professor. "I cooperatively traveled to where I was directed and went through whatever tests were requested of me."

Despite his undergoing a large number of additional laboratory and clinical examinations, including a PSA test, serum chemistry profiles, bone chemistry enzymes, carcinoembryonic antigen (CEA), chest X-rays, CT scan of the lower abdomen, and urological ultrasound to measure tumor size, no dramatic treatment was recommended or administered for his prostate cancer.

"Let's give no treatment but rather watch the tumor and observe its growth," was the decision agreed upon by Dr. Henri Boiteux's country urologist in conjunction with another urologist and a prostate gland specialist his personal doctor had called in as consultants.

Prostate cancer is the second most common cause of cancer death among men worldwide, in particular throughout Europe and the United States. (Lung cancer is the most frequent source of malignancy death for both men and women.) When prostatic tissue is examined microscopically, cancer is found in 50 percent of men over age seventy, and it's present in virtually all men over ninety. Most of the time such cancers never cause symptoms, but 3 percent of men exhibiting diseased prostate tissue die of it.[49]

There are a number of invasive treatment options; most of them poor. For example, world-class golf professional Arnold Palmer was diagnosed with prostate cancer which remained confined to the one organ and was not metastatic. The golfer underwent a radical prostatectomy (complete surgical removal of his prostate) at the Mayo Clinic in Rochester, Minnesota. But some weeks later it was revealed that the initial therapy selected had been inappropriate and ineffective for him since Mr. Palmer required follow up radiation. Thus the Mayo Clinic, known for its urologic excellence and care and attended by supposedly the world's most brilliant minds and skilled surgeons, had rendered flawed treatment to Arnold Palmer's diseased organ. Such inappropriate therapy is common for the diseased prostate.

In a normal adult man under age thirty-five, the prostate weighs about twenty grams, but thereafter, it tends to generally increase in size. Above fifty grams the gland is considered "enlarged" and urologists call this Benign Prostatic Hyperplasia (BPH).[50]

"Prostate cancer is always found together with prostatitis and all men will probably get both diseases if they live long enough," says urological surgeon Ronald E. Wheeler, M.D., Medical Director of the Diagnostic Center for Disease in Sarasota, Florida. Dr. Wheeler adds, "It is time to rethink how we handle prostate cancer."[51]

When Dr. Boiteux showed an elevated Prostate Specific Antigen (PSA), he received an initial ultrasound examination which also revealed a suspicious hard nodule inside his prostate gland. His biopsy, taken under local anesthesia, was subjected to biochemical and histological tests (a microscopic analysis of the prostate tissue) which determined that the gland's growth was of a nonaggressive type of cancer. It had not metastasized. The former physics professor was lucky in that he was not in immediate danger, but his prostate diagnosis was reconfirmed as a definite cancer when he underwent still another biopsy.

Professor Boiteux was diagnosed with prostate cancer nine years before I interviewed him in September 2003. Before using Beljanski's supplements, he tried the conventional route. To treat the man's life-threatening illness, the medical consultants from Paris who had been called in to examine him offered no recommendations to the patient's personal urologist except to watch and wait. However, Boiteux's uncertain country urologist finally decided to do something on his own. He elected to supervise, from a distance, the use of cancer-corrective hormonal treatment. Henri Boiteux received hormone-diminishing treatment from an endocrine gland therapist at a sophisticated hospital clinic in Paris throughout July 1994. The country urologist kept apprised of his progress—or lack of it.

The patient took the approved quantity of anti-hormone substances for several months but with no observable result. He grew discouraged, subsequently stopped the anti-hormonal medications, and remained in Paris. Professor Boiteux did not return to his country home in the South of France until after the first of August 1994. It was then that a long-time close personal friend—another well-respected former university professor—visited him. This gentleman was somewhat knowledgeable about holistic adjunctive treatment for malignant tumors. He knew a number of doctors who administered them.

"My visitor told me," continued Dr. Boiteux, "'since you've advised me that you eventually may be forced to take radiotherapy for your prostate, I recommend that you consult a medical doctor I know, who utilizes certain complementary treatment products in his cancer practice. He is providing excellent results for patients just like you. Possibly this physician will help you to overcome the negative side effects that invariably accompany radiation treatment.'"

"I was open to my friend's suggestion," Boiteux asserted.

Professor Boiteux followed his colleague's advice and consulted this recommended therapist who practices CAIM (Complementary, Alternative, and Integrative Medicine). Dr. Philippe Causé, M.D., thinks holistically, administering natural and non-toxic therapies to his patients. The French holistic physician subsequently dispensed two of Dr. Mirko Beljanski's anticancer herbal supplements to Professor Henri Boiteux, for Dr. Causé's experience was that they had worked effectively against cancers of several types before. His patients had benefited repeatedly. "I use Dr. Beljanski's supplements as therapeutic preventatives," Dr. Causé told the professor.

Professor Boiteux was given golden-leaf *Ginkgo biloba* extract as well as the herbal alkaloid of Pao pereira. He ingested the two products faithfully and within a very short time the frequency of urinary urgency reduced from up to six times per night to just three. But while the urgency to urinate diminished, he was sometimes unable to bring on a urine stream. And once per week he found that his urine contained bright red blood. Men with prostate disease are likely to identify with these same prostatic difficulties as the professor. But within a month to six weeks, with the ingestion of two of Beljanski's products, dispensed to him by Dr. Causé, all of his prostatic disease signs and symptoms improved. Dr. Boiteux continued to ingest the anticancer botanicals that Dr. Causé had prescribed.

After another six months of using Beljanski's products, having long since discontinued the anti-hormonal therapy and still never having received radiotherapy, Professor Boiteux again traveled to Paris for a third full series of physical and laboratory examinations. These reports from the hospital clinic's radiology and oncology departments and from the on-staff urologists who examined him were that Dr. Boiteux's prostate cancer was regressing—the enlarged gland itself had shrunk to less than half its original pathological size. These observing hospital doctors were confused and then upset by their inability to explain any reason for this man's improvement, and they reported this to both the patient and to the patient's country urologist.

"Don't Tell Me About Beljanski!"

With great joy Professor Boiteux reported to the Parisian hospital specialists first and then to his urologist in the south of France that the healing progress shown by the internal organ's rejection of malignancy was likely coming from his ingestion of Beljanski's supplements. They were the only pills he had been taking routinely. The hospital-based consultants listened and shrugged their shoulders with no verbal comment.

Despite being his personal urologist, the country specialist, however, appeared most irritated and even was aggressive in his response to the news. He literally shouted at Henri Boiteux, "I know about Beljanski, and I don't want to hear anything more about him or his therapy. He is practicing medicine without a license. So don't tell me about Beljanski!" The doctor then stormed out of the consultation room of his country office, and Professor Boiteux sat there for a long time in a state of shock.

In about twenty minutes, the urologist returned and handed his patient a written prescription to take to a pharmacist. It contained nothing related to Beljanski's products; instead, it was another prescription for anti-hormonal medications, which Professor Boiteux had previously received and not filled. The pharmaceutical order also held no mention of radiotherapy. His country urologist additionally told Professor Boiteux, "You can take anything else that you want, but I don't want to hear about how you are treating yourself. If there is something more that you want to swallow, you are free to do that, but do not tell me."

In effect, Professor Boiteux was on his own, for he did not take any of the anti-hormone medications and continued with Beljanski's products. By May 1995 the prostate pathology had completely disappeared and his PSA was down from 9.6 ng/ml to essentially normal at 4.0 ng/ml. The patient felt happy beyond words.

Six months later, he became overly confident in his body's new-found health. The Professor told me, "I asked myself—being a man of science specializing in physics—what has cured me? I decided to stop taking these two Beljanski products just to see what would happen. Whether or not he wanted to hear from me or about Beljanskis work, I wrote to my local country urologist and made him an offer. I told him that he could use me as a human guinea pig to see if the prostate cancer would return as a result of my discontinuing the ingestion of Beljanski's two herbs."

"My doctor wrote back two weeks later and did not mention the Beljanski herbal products. Instead he issued me a warning, saying: 'When prostate cancer returns after it has been in remission, it is twice as difficult to treat and get rid of a second time.' I understood his warning and was cautioned by it," Professor Boiteux said.

One of Beljanski's Herbals Helps Osteoarthritic Knee Pain

The professor continued: "Then one evening about six weeks later as I was preparing to take a shower, arthritic-type pains hit me once again in both knees. Perhaps I failed to mention to you the osteoarthritis that had been bothering me for more than twelve years stopped causing me any difficulty when I began to take Beljanski's supplements. After I had taken Dr. Beljanski's herbal extracts, the pains disappeared and I hadn't experienced pains in my knees for at least a year. In fact, I had forgotten about these osteoarthritic joint pains, as I had become much more concerned about the prostate cancer, which was of course more serious.

"The resumption of my previous osteoarthritic symptoms was taken by me as a message that at least one of Dr. Beljanski's products had to become part of my life once again. I didn't resume taking the *Ginkgo biloba* because it had been dispensed to me by Dr. Philippe Causé specifically to neutralize the negative effects of radiotherapy, which Dr. Causé assumed I would take; but I had not received any radiation. So I restarted only the Pao pereira herbal extract at a somewhat lower dosage from six capsules daily to four capsules daily.

"The knee pains went away fast, but when I reduced the dosage a few months later to just three capsules per day, the arthritic pains returned. Four Pao pereira was better for me—if I continued to take two in the morning and two at night, my arthritic knees gave me no problems. As I've stated, I did not resume taking the *Ginkgo biloba* at all," says Dr. Boiteux. "As far as my mind, emotions and body are concerned, I am feeling alert, relaxed, vigorous, strong and fine in every way—a state of health that I attribute to my use of Dr. Mirko Beljanski's herbal extracts."

Professor Boiteux also made it very clear that he wished to add this final observation to my report on his case study: "As a man of science, I believe I'm qualified to make a certain judgment. My declaration is that the readers of your book, Dr. Walker, will come to recognize this truth: Dr. Mirko Beljanski's intellectual prowess combined the experimental curiosity of Michael Faraday [the father of modern electrical theory], the methodical rigor of Antoine Lavoisier [the father of modern chemistry], the theoretical vision of Albert Einstein [the father of modern physics], and the inventive genius of Thomas Edison [the father of modern technological innovation]."

I couldn't agree more.

5

Integrative Cancer Therapy: The Power of Combining Alternative With Conventional

When you or someone you love is told "you have cancer," I'm certain the response is universal—I know I felt it. Fear grips your gut, and you're sent into an emotional tailspin. Most likely the first thing you're going to ask the doctor is "what are my chances?" The answers will range from being really good to facing death in a few weeks or months. It's a terribly draining experience.

One thing is for certain. When you are told you have cancer, you know you are soon to be making some hard choices in terms of treatment. The doctors most likely will push for conventional treatment, but if you've done your homework, you might not be so willing to go that discouraging route. You think about trying alternative treatments, or perhaps you're a die-hard like me, and you would never even consider doing chemo or radiation.

Treatment decisions are difficult. Cancer is a disease that has defied every conventional and most alternative therapies thrown at it. Sometimes some drug or herb works, sometimes it doesn't. Sometimes the cancer comes back, other times it stays in remission forever.

Fortunately, it is becoming more and more common for cancer patients to choose a balance between the worlds of holistic and conventional cancer treatments. While the two medical philosophies differ markedly, research shows that combined they can be extraordinarily effective.

Together they are called complementary or integrative therapy. It is not something that is standardized or even yet widely accepted; each doctor you talk to will probably have a different idea of what integrative therapy is. According to the clinical journal, *Integrative Cancer Therapies* (*ICT*), integrative therapy is the "scientific understanding of alternative medicine and traditional medicine therapies, and their responsible integration with conventional health care. Integrative care includes therapeutic interventions in diet, lifestyle, exercise, stress care, and nutritional supplements, as well as experimental vaccines, chrono-chemotherapy [adapting chemotherapy to your natural rhythm of sleep and awake time], and other advanced treatments." [52]

Integrative therapy is the wave of the future in cancer treatments, but it is definitely a "consumer beware" situation. There are those who are already abusing the idea by merely giving nod to alternative treatments. They are privileging conventional chemo and radiation therapy while vilifying the nutritional supplement aspect of integration—most likely as a way to appease Big Pharma while appearing to be participating in the new game of integration. One notable doctor, Aaron Katz, M.D., Director for the Center for Holistic Urology, takes the idea of integration seriously.

The mission of the Center for Holistic Urology (CHU) echoes the definition of the journal noted above. It includes complementary therapies such as acupuncture, clinical nutrition, botanical medicine, exercise and mind-body therapies, and its goal is to "promote wider knowledge and understanding of such therapies by conducting high-quality basic science research and clinical trials." [53]

So what do we have to lose? There are roughly half-a-million cancer patients who will die in the U.S. alone by the end of this year and another seven million more people around the globe.[54] Over 11,700,000 are living with the disease right now and nearly all of them know it. More, of course, will be diagnosed next year.

But here's the question we all have to ask ourselves: does it really matter how you kill cancer cells as long as they are dead?

Proven Synergy with Chemotherapeutic Agents

When I embarked on my mission, I wanted to make Dr. Beljanski's botanicals the alternative cancer resource of choice. I would still love for that to happen, but I have also come to respect the microbiologist and what he stood for. As Melissa Burchill, the dietician nutritionist who wrote up the results of the Columbia clinical trials of the bolt molecules, succinctly put it, "Patients should bear in mind that Dr. Beljanski conceived of these plant extracts as adjuncts to conventional cancer treatment."[55] Dr. Beljanski never wanted to buck the conventional trend. Rather, he was integrative from the beginning, constantly searching for ways to make conventional medical treatments more effective.

When I first started studying Beljanski's work, I could barely contain my excitement as I realized how thoroughly he researched every aspect of DNA destabilization and the botanicals to correct the problem. Dr. Beljanski's approach to what causes cancer as well as the two bolt molecules that can kill the cancerous cell has some serious science behind it; he has 133 refereed publications to his name. (In the world of science and academia, refereed means that one's work is reviewed by one's peers before it is put into publication.)

But it was one of the later studies, the one I noted in the preface, that electrified me to my core. Dr. Beljanski, towards the end of his life, asked another "what if" question—what would happen if he paired his botanicals with conventional chemo and radiation? The results were stunning: chemo and radiation were markedly more effective when used in conjunction with the anticancer botanicals of Pao pereira and *R. vomitoria*.

Cancer Cells 100 Percent Dead

In order to answer his question of whether or not conventional treatments would be enhanced by the bolt molecules, he first had to test the substances in test tubes. When that showed promising results, he knew not to get excited. Within all organisms, any drug faces a complicated array of physiological regulations. Some will contribute to the elimination of the drug before it has had time to act; others will just simply resist the drug's effect. Compounds which are introduced at high levels of dosage with food may not be absorbed sufficiently because something in the food interferes with the absorption of the drug. In addition, each individual's biochemistry is unique and great variations exist from person to person in terms of how a drug is handled, metabolized, and eliminated. Such countless interactions are the real stumbling blocks for optimal action by any medication introduced into the organism. For this reason, agents that appear to work *in vitro* may result in disappointing results, and even no results, *in vivo*. This, however, was not the case with the two Beljanski herbal extracts.

Beljanski and his team found in a series of trials in mice, that they could, under certain circumstances, produce the previously unheard of result of *100 percent cured*.

I also had to chuckle with satisfaction, for once I understood the science—in typical Beljanski fashion—it made perfectly logical sense and presented the ultimate in integrative science.

It really was quite simple. In an attempt to improve the treatment results in those mice receiving *in vivo* transplanted cancers, Beljanski combined his plant extracts with a low dosage of conventional chemotherapeutic cytotoxic (cell-killing) agents.

Beljanski reasoned that in low dosages, cytotoxic agents and/or radiotherapy would destabilize cancerous DNA. Yes, this action does cause more cancerous damage, but that was precisely the point. Any carcinogen keeps the replicated DNA strand from closing up, thereby causing it to duplicate itself *ad infinitum*. Cancer-killing agents, working as carcinogens, lay open additional strands of DNA which allows the bolt molecule to better penetrate the cancerous cell, thereby allowing the botanicals to do their job even more effectively.

In other words, chemotherapy and radiation are in essence the sucker punch that allows the knockout blow to happen.

The results were excellent for his cancer-ridden laboratory animals. The rate of improvement when the botanicals were combined with the cytotoxic agent was far more effective than using either one alone.

Then, to further demonstrate the advantage of combining the two types of treatment, a series of experiments were undertaken on mice with a naturally developed and highly dangerous strand of lymphoma (technically labeled YC-8), a permanent cancer of the lymphatic vessels in mammals. The lymphoma test was in contrast to most of the other experiments, which involved transplantable cancers such as splicing breast cancer cells straight into the laboratory animal.

The mice for this study were divided into four groups:

- One group received no treatment. This was the control group.

- The second group received only low doses of the chemotherapeutic agent.

- The third group received only Beljanski's *Rauwolfia vomitoria* extract.

- The fourth group received a combination of the low dose chemotherapy and the *Rauwolfia* botanical.

The result?

The control animals receiving no treatment were all dead from cancer invasion by the thirtieth day—no survival.

The survival rate for the second cancerous group (mice treated only with the chemotherapeutic agent CCNU) at ninety days was 45 percent.

The survival rate for those cancer-filled mice treated with only the *Rauwolfia* extract at ninety days was 30 percent.

But in the fourth cancerous group, when the two treatments were combined (the extract plus the CCNU), Beljanski's team found that one, the tumor did not have a chance to develop significantly (which was what happened in the other three groups), and two, the mouse survival rate reached an *unexpected high of 100 percent.*[56]

This kind of result is practically unheard of in any study on cancer cells and anticancer remedies, natural or synthetic.

Other similar tests were conducted combining the alkaloids with additional cytotoxics standardly used in human chemotherapy. The results recorded were all exceedingly positive. Those mice receiving the low dose chemotherapy along with Dr. Beljanski's botanicals generally survived their cancers. Those receiving chemotherapy alone did not!

And again, the Beljanski team found that both anticancer alkaloid extracts are selective; they attach only to cancerous DNA and do not affect normal and healthy DNA nor any other part of a viable cell. In test after test, the laboratory animals that were affected by cancer but recovered survived for prolonged periods and remained in excellent health. They suffered neither from weight loss nor other undesirable side effects. These extracts prevented the synthetic and toxic chemotherapy as well as the radiotherapy from producing their usual harmful effects.

Beljanski showed during the decade of the 1980s—a dramatic and true medical breakthrough—that a cure for cancer *in vivo* is available.

All experiments conducted by Dr. Beljanski were replicated multiple times using both alkaloids and various methods of administration: oral, intravenous, intra-peritoneal (directly into the body cavity), and intralesionally (directly into the tumor). It was thanks to the French Army, that the integrative effect of the bolt molecules with both chemotherapy and radiation therapy could be exploited. Because of his contract with the army, Beljanski's research team had the resources for experimentation, access to gamma radiation, and massive amounts of laboratory mice to use in experiments.

Here again, this is a study that needs to be repeated in American laboratories to confirm the results. But as a long-time proponent of alternative therapies, I was truly awed to learn that Beljanski would even consider doing a study combining his bolt molecules with conventional cancer treatments. I was even more excited—and humbled—by the excellent responses the integrative approach had against cancer.

RNA Fragments—Integrative Approach #2

That study made me revisit Beljanski's early work on RNA and radiation to find if this trend of integration had started earlier, and if so when. (RNA is the other nucleic acid in the cell and it plays a critical role in helping DNA do its work as well as transporting material around the cell. RNA also has a number of independent functions which are no less important than DNA.) What I found was that Beljanski had been integrative from the beginning, for he discovered, during the course of his life-time at the laboratory bench, two other substances that enhanced the effects of the traditional treatments: one made from RNA fragments; the other coming not from the green but from the golden leaf of the ancient and remarkably resilient *Ginkgo biloba* tree. Beljanski discovered that these two substances helped the body recover from the nasty side effects of conventional treatment, so much so in some cases that the chemo or radiation could be continued for longer periods and even higher doses, thereby killing more cancer cells.

Early Research on RNA

Dr. Mirko Beljanski spent the bulk of his professional life devoted not to cancerous DNA but to uncovering the mysteries of RNA. I have related the story of Beljanski's discoveries concerning cancerous DNA first because I feel they rank above RNA in importance in the real war against cancer. However, the DNA research, as you have seen by the dates I gave you, came later in Beljanski's career. The thirty years he spent at the Pasteur Institute, from 1948 to 1978, were dedicated to some of the earliest discoveries in modern research on RNA and its relationship to DNA.

His interest in RNA was at direct odds with the Institute's director Jacques Monod, Ph.D. Dr. Monod declared that everyone under his employ was to work on the "central dogma" of DNA and accept RNA simply as its "messenger boy." [57] Beljanski ignored his boss and made some of the most important discoveries of his career with RNA, such as the role of RNA is as fundamental as DNA in terms of cell duplication and protein synthesis. Proteins, as I mentioned in chapter 1, are essential for one's total physiology because protein is required basically for everything having to do with the physical body: the structure, function, and regulation of the body's cells, tissues, and organs. Protein synthesis, then, is vital for life to continue.

Beljanski is also arguably the first to have discovered the enzyme "reverse transcriptase"—so named because it reverses the usual transcription of DNA into RNA. In order for genetic information to be passed from DNA to the rest of the cell and hence to the body as a whole, it has to be transferred from DNA into RNA. Reverse transcription means that RNA is actually transferring genetic information into DNA—the reverse of the usual process. Reverse transcription has become important to all of humanity because of the HIV virus that works exactly on that principle. It is a very complex process, but the simple effect of it is that it enables a virus to be inserted into the host's DNA and replicated by the host and that's why HIV seems impossible to cure or even treat with any good effect. [58]

Dr. Beljanski was definitely the first to detect reverse transcriptase in bacteria in 1974. Dr. James Grutsch, clinical-trial consultant to the Cancer Treatment Centers of America, who was a fledgling scientist at the Pasteur Institute during Beljanski's term there, elegantly explains, "Dr. Beljanski was pioneering research into [RNA] and proving RNA indeed spoke back to DNA and gave it new information that changed its [DNA's] blueprint." Dr. Grutsch, nodding to the constant dissention between Beljanski and Monod, adds, "If [Beljanski] survived all those years under a director like Monod—who did not tolerate dummies— he must have been a darn good scientist. He had done all of the work to show us that we could actually save lives with RNA." [59]

Because Dr. Beljanski's research into RNA is so extensive and quite scientifically complicated, I am not going to go into detail here. But if you're interested in acquiring further information, please see *A Pioneer in Biomedicine* by C.G. Nordau and Monique Beljanski; *Extraordinary Healing* by L. Stephen Coles, M.D., Ph.D.; and the numbers of pertinent publications listed in Appendix B authored or coauthored by Mirko Beljanski in which you can learn more about Dr. Beljanski's important discoveries in RNA.

For our purposes, what Beljanski discovered concerning RNA will make chemotherapy or radiotherapy patients rejoice, for they will no longer need to experience its extensive complications or other adverse side effects! That alone makes Beljanski's discoveries good candidates to be included in the acceptable integrative treatments used in forward-thinking cancer hospitals around the world.

Primer RNA

RNA comes in many forms in every human cell, and it plays a central part in the cell's ability to replicate itself. Some of the common forms of RNA that you might come across are *messenger RNA* (mRNA). This is what RNA is most known for. This is the type of RNA that tells the cell what genetic message is being transferred from the DNA.

Next there is *transfer RNA* (tRNA). It takes the genetic information and transfers it to the rest of the cell, so that the cell knows what kind of protein it needs to make. When I talked about protein composition in chapter 1, I talked about how amino acids are bonded together with peptides to form the polypeptide chains of protein. Transfer RNA brings the correct amino acids to the ribosome in a cell. A ribosome is the part of a cell that manufactures protein, which brings us to another type of RNA, what microbiologists have identified as *ribosomal RNA* (rRNA).

Ribosomal RNA is the molecular component of a ribosome. Some biochemists have called it the "cell's essential protein factory"[60] because rRNA actually fabricates the polypeptides that bond the amino acids together. The importance of RNA to the functioning of our bodies at the cellular structure cannot be discounted. It's everything! Without it we are nothing, literally no muscles, no tissues, no organs—all those things that hold our bodies together.

After Beljanski detected reverse transcriptase in bacteria in 1974, he asked himself in his daily journal: "Would promoting DNA in the bone marrow facilitate the appearance of blood cells?"

His answer led him to find a technique to produce something called small primer RNA's. "Small" RNA are so called because they are non-coding, meaning they don't translate into a protein molecule. "Primer" means that they prepare the site of the DNA strand that is be replicated. With his young and enthusiastic apprentice, Michel Plawecki, Ph.D., Dr. Beljanski was able to find an RNA primer that would be specific to enhancing DNA synthesis of mammalian bone marrow.

He produced the primer from ribosomal RNA, but he had to figure out how to first isolate rRNA and then "cleave" it or cut it up with pancreatic enzymes. With this process, he had discovered yet another monumental way to help all those who suffered the severe side effects of conventional cancer treatments.

In order to ensure that their primer was as close to physiologically produced ones as possible, the two biological scientists prepared RNA fragments from rRNA using the RNA from safe-origin bacteria *E. coli* K12, a natural host in the human intestinal track and well-known to be harmless. The RNA fragments are made from an extract of *E. coli* K-12 bacteria that has been purified repeatedly so it is very safe for human consumption. They then split or "cleaved" the rRNA by the pancreatic enzyme I mentioned above, creating their RNA fragments.

These fragments they found behaved like selective promoters of bone marrow DNA. Bone marrow is where blood cells, both white and red, plus the platelets are manufactured.

Platelets are irregularly shaped, colorless bodies in the blood that help it form clots. When the platelet count is too low, excessive bleeding can occur. White blood cells, also called leukocytes, are the cells in the blood that help the body defend itself against both infectious disease and foreign materials. Red blood cells are a bit more resistant to chemo and radiation, but there are some chemotherapy drugs that attack those as well. A low count of red blood cells means that your body isn't getting enough oxygen, for the red blood cells are responsible for transporting that very essential element from your lungs to the rest of your body.

It is a work-intensive process to procure the RNA fragments, but Beljanski proved they could help bone marrow stem cells speed up the production of both red and white blood cells and platelets. Just as important, the bacterial RNA fragments did not act on the *in vivo* brain, lungs, or muscles, nor on leukemia cells. When injected into living animals, these fragments concentrated on the spleen and the bone marrow of the animal, which was a good sign.

Knowledge about this is tremendously important for patients undergoing chemotherapy. One of the unwanted side effects of taking cytotoxic chemicals to kill cancer is that it attacks the body's healthy bone marrow, gastrointestinal tract, and the mouth. Mucous membranes in the mouth, for instance, split, crack, and cause burning as a result of chemotherapy, but this can be alleviated or prevented altogether by the use of RNA primers.[61]

RNA Primers Stimulate Blood Cells *In vivo*

After Beljanski's team affirmed RNA fragments promote blood-cell production in bone marrow *in vitro*, they proceeded to the next phase, testing the substance on rabbits. Healthy rabbits were given high doses of antimitotics (a type of chemotherapy in which drugs help stop the cell from dividing and thus act as anti-tumor agents). Without ingesting RNA fragments, the animals would have died within ten days from the cell-killing effects of the antimitotics because of the very high dosage given. The blood cells were measured every day. Each time the animals received RNA fragments following a drop in blood cells, their cell counts reflected an immediate increase in white blood cells and platelets.

Results from the administration of RNA fragments were usually obtained within forty-eight hours. At that time during the ten-year period starting from 1975, the RNA fragments were given by injection. Now they are administered orally, and studies show they do provide excellent results both for restoration of white blood cells and platelets. These fragments bring about little effect on red blood cells whose maturation cycle is much longer.[62]

Of particular interest in this discussion of integrative cancer therapies is the Beljanski team's observation that the RNA fragments from the purified strain of *E. coli* fight the *imbalance* that chemotherapeutic drugs, especially the antimitotics, induce in various cell lines that ordinarily produce white blood cells. In the presence of chemotherapeutic drugs, white cells with many nuclei (called polynuclear leucocytes) which are largely responsible for defense against infection, disappeared faster than the lymphocytes, the smaller white blood cells associated with the lymphatic system, thus creating an unwanted imbalance. The RNA fragments restored the imbalance induced by the toxic treatments, thus allowing the chemotherapy or radiotherapy to work more effectively. And, like the two anticancer botanicals, it also proved to be selective, for it only stimulates the growth of healthy white blood cells and platelets.

Platelet Counts are Restored

Chemotherapy can also create a condition known as thrombocytopenia, where the blood platelet counts drop to dangerously low levels. The problem with your blood-cell count and/or your platelet count dipping too low is that the chemical or radiation treatments must stop because you could either bleed to death or be killed during the course of being treated by an otherwise curable disease. But stopping treatment leaves the body vulnerable to the cancer cells resuming their unceasing replication—a condition no cancer patient wants.

While hospitals now regularly use synthetic medicines to help boost the production of white blood cells, until Beljanski's research was rediscovered, there was nothing natural to help the blood-cell dilemma and nothing at all to help increase platelet count except to stop treatment and give a blood transfusion.

Beljanski and his team found that the RNA fragments promoted the quick appearance of new platelets to replace the platelets destroyed by chemotherapy. More importantly, the repeated doses of these fragments did not lead to tolerance or toxicity among cancer-affected rabbits treated with the antimitotics that are so toxic to healthy cells. Increased dosage was without incidence since the fragments were found to be destroyed within four hours by means of various enzymes in the blood that dissolve the nucleic acids in water so that they can be flushed from the body. What's more, they did not block the action of the antimitotics and could be applied with almost any cancer-fighting agent.

After uncovering the restorative effects of RNA fragments *in vivo*, the microbiologist teamed up with several M.D.s who administered the fragments to people with cancer. The RNA fragments behaved the same in humans as they did *in vivo*, protecting patients receiving radiation therapy and intensive chemotherapy. This was a new beneficial situation which worked well, provided that human patients received enough RNA primers early in their conventional treatments. Beljanski found the primers need to be ingested before all of the cancer patient's bone marrow stem cells are destroyed by chemotherapeutic poisons. [63]

However, the evidence is clear: RNA fragments, priming only healthy cells, are powerful healing agents. The other rare cases where RNA fragments show no effect against the side effects of cancer are either when there is a lack of hemoglobin (in red blood cells which number less than 2.5 million) or when there is an excess of ribonuclease in the blood (ribonuclease is an important enzyme that breaks down RNA into smaller components in part to help the body get rid of excess RNA), which may be partially inhibited by the ingestion of magnesium. An excess in ferritin (a mineral component in which iron is linked to a protein) can also slow down RNA fragment activity.

Recent Clinical Trials of RNA Fragments

Dr. Michael Schachter firmly believes that cancer victims and other people receiving chemotherapy could benefit from taking RNA fragments.[64] There are some pioneers in cancer research who believe as Dr. Schachter does and are taking the study of RNA fragments a step further by initiating clinical trials as the means to instill confidence in this non-toxic but experimental approach. In early 2005, a Phase I clinical trial focusing on RNA fragments was initiated at the Cancer Treatment Centers of America (CTCA). The Center's trial was titled "Study on the role of an RNA-fragment-based dietary supplement in the maintenance of white blood cell production during chemotherapy." The chemotherapy protocol these patients underwent was extremely heavy, and they were particularly at risk of hemorrhage following the loss of their platelets. By using RNA-fragments, patients in the CTCA clinical trial avoided such risks. Further clinical trials began again in January of 2008.

In 2010, Drs. Levin, Daehler, Grutsch, Hall, Gupta, and Lis reported the findings of those trials. The trials were conducted as an onsite study at the Cancer Treatment Centers of America at Midwestern Regional Medical Center in Zion, Illinois. Thirty-two patients underwent a clinical trial using these RNA fragments of the *E. coli* bacteria. Forty different patients signed a consent form to participate in a separate trial using RNA fragments derived from yeast. The trial was set up to study platelet counts in patients who had varying degrees of exposure to chemotherapy to see which RNA fragments—the yeast-derived or the *E coli*-derived—

were more effective. Twenty-four of the patients had in fact previously failed between one to nine prior regiments.

The results of the study were striking. The researchers state, "The primary goal of anti-chemotherapy induced thrombocytopenia (when platelets are lost from the bloodstream faster than they can be replaced) is the avoidance of delays in treatment and reductions in the dose of chemotherapy. Four patients experienced a treatment delay or reduction in chemotherapy dosage in the yeast-fragment arm of the trial, but *no* patient using *E. coli* RNA fragments had an unplanned dose reduction or delay" (proving that not all RNA fragments are created equal). They further state that at the higher dosage level of sixty or eighty milligrams of the *E. coli* RNA fragments, there were no platelet transfusions required.

The researchers conclude that "at all doses, patients receiving *E. coli* RNA fragments showed a recovery in platelet numbers of 80,000/ml by the end of eight days following chemotherapy nadir (the low point of the platelet count)" and, given the data found in the study, the CTCA plans "further clinical trials designed to measure the efficacy of *E. coli* RNA fragments in the management of Chemotherapy-induced Thrombocytopenia (CIT) among patients with advanced cancer."

Similar comments to those of the CTCA were made by Maurice Stroun, Ph.D., Professor of Biochemistry at Switzerland's University of Geneva. I conducted a one-on-one tape-recorded interview of Dr. Stroun in Paris when he visited with me on September 6, 2003. Dr. Stroun enthusiastically praised the anticancer research of Mirko Beljanski. As part of his statement, he made some personal remarks. Among them he said:

"Right now, there's only one real supplement for the adverse effects of chemotherapy and radiation therapy, and that's RNA fragments. I have a friend who recently had a serious case of leukemia…thanks to the RNA fragments, he was able to request heavier chemotherapy than is normally given and to significantly increase his chances of survival. The product definitely has that effect. And the fact that it doesn't have any side effects—that's what's really fantastic!"

Dr. James F. Grutsch has provided the definitive word on the utter applicability of these RNA fragments: he considers this "concentrated source" of RNA a "food." He states, "RNA fragments can be essential nutrients…Every time you eat salads or meat, you are eating RNA." He adds that while other products proclaim to maintain healthy platelet counts, "they do not. There is something about what Beljanski specifically uncovered that is completely unique." [66]

RNA fragments are practically always active. Because of their specific action on bone marrow, they make it possible to see a rise in white blood cell and platelet blood count levels within forty-eight hours. The stability, user-friendliness and effectiveness of RNA fragments are, indeed, physiologically remarkable.

Moreover, the idea behind the creation of RNA fragments was completely original. It opens the door to new perspectives on the selective activation of certain genes, which could lead to a completely novel therapeutic approach to cancer. The fact that they are not transcribed in DNA, that they only prime or prepare one's physiology for a single action, and that afterwards they are broken down and eliminated by plasma nucleases, all create a powerful argument in favor of their safety.

I have already emphasized in terms of the anticancer molecules from Pao pereira and *Rauwolfia vomitoria* that *selectivity* is an idea which should be the cornerstone for the next generation of non-toxic and natural therapeutic products from plants, from microorganisms, and/or from animals. This development of *E. coli* RNA fragments represents one of Dr. Mirko Beljanski's greatest conceptual advancements, and it should stand as a cornerstone in integrative cancer therapies now and in the future.

Ginkgo biloba—Integrative Approach #3

Up to this point, we have talked mostly about chemotherapy and the toxic side effects it has on the human body. I have mentioned radiotherapy throughout, but have not addressed it directly up until this point. Radiation treatment has long been used to fight cancer. It is supposed to shrink tumors by killing the cancer cells.

Radiation is also a known carcinogen. People everywhere are talking about radiation and the danger X-rays, high tension wires, computer screens, microwaves, mammographies, scans, airport screens, cell phones, iPhones, and the myriad of other electronic devices we're attached to practically all the time. Such conveniences unquestionably pose dangers to our chromosomes. They are a main underlying source of the increase in cancer found in every population in the civilized world.

Radiation exposes all persons to measurable and immeasurable harm. Several highly critical articles, written by specialists on these issues, can be found on the internet. For example, J.W. Gofman, Ph.D., Professor Emeritus of Molecular and Cellular Biology at the University of California, Berkeley—not one to talk about a subject of which he is unaware—led a massive investigation involving scientists, doctors, etiologists (the scientists who study the origins and causes of disease) and physicians. The investigation was published in November 1999. The investigators concluded, in print, some crystal-clear truths. According to Dr. Gofman's research, medical radiation, introduced as a treatment in 1896, is becoming a factor in approximately half of all fatal cases of cancer in the U.S. The proof cited in his 1999 monograph, which no one has refuted, indicates that approximately two-hundred fifty thousand people in the U.S. die prematurely each year from cancer and coronary diseases, with half the cases due to the unnecessary and excessive use of X-rays that they received over a lifetime. [67]

The warning is clear: minimize or avoid any exposure to X-rays of any kind. Radiation due to medical imaging is the underlying causative factor in approximately half of the fatalities in the treatment of coronary diseases in the U.S. Also, with the inappropriate use of CT Scans, MRIs, SPECT Scans, and other forms of medical imaging, danger lies waiting in everyone's future. Due to concern for profitability, negligence, and lack of coordination, medical imaging is overused and is administered at excessive doses. Remember, I am still only talking about medical imaging, to say nothing of therapeutic radiation treatments for cancer.

Since risks associated with radiation are cumulative and proportional to accumulated doses of X-rays, one should (and can) insist that our doctors and radiologists reduce by half regular doses administered in radiation therapy, scans, fluoroscopes, etc. In other words, beware of diagnostic X-rays.

Dangers from Diagnostic Radiation and Radiotherapy

It is well known that some of the conventional oncological treatments, particularly radiation therapy, can induce DNA mutations, fibrosis, or smoldering skin burns. The lowered immunity in scar tissue predisposes it to what's called malignant degeneration, the transformation of a benign lesion anywhere in the body into a malignant one. According to research oncologist, Dr. E. B. Kaplan: "There is an elevated mortality rate: one out of three or four patients with burns or osteomyelitis (a bone infection), or irradiated cancer dies from dermatological complications." [68]

The dangers to which I am referring relate to both diagnostic radiation and radiotherapy. They fall into two categories of damage to human beings:

a. DNA breakages and mutations

b. Alteration in the DNA's secondary structure (DNA destabilization)

A main goal in Dr. Mirko Beljanski's research, which was evidenced in the improvement experienced by patients undergoing chemotherapy, radiation therapy, and other harsh treatments, was prevention of unhealthy cell multiplication. His major goal, always, was to improve a patient's chances for homeostasis, the ideal state of the body by which all systems maintain a stable, constant condition.

You have just read about the ability of RNA fragments to handle dangerously low white blood cell and platelet counts. Dr. Mirko Beljanski and his team also discovered in the late 1970s that a particular variation of the leaf from the *Ginkgo biloba* tree can be used to handle the myriad of side effects of radiation (as well as surgery) including burns, fibrosis, and the normalization of abnormal proteins.

Studies in Radiation Poisoning

On March 17, 1978, Dr. Mirko Beljanski and his wife were no longer allowed access to the laboratories at the Pasteur Institute. As I reported in the previous chapter, upon expulsion from the Pasteur, they found a new home for their microbiological investigations at France's Châtenay-Malabry School of Pharmacy. [69] There, the Beljanskis were awarded the six-year contract with the French army I mentioned above to study phenomena involved in protecting against radiation. Beljanski and his student-turned-colleague, Dr. Michel Plawecki, were able to study at length both the effects of various doses of gamma rays on rabbits and mice as well as certain substances able to protect, to some degree, the organs of irradiated laboratory animals. In particular, he researched how these animals could be shielded from the damage and alterations engendered by radiation-derived toxicity.

Radiation induces body burns inside and outside. In particular it brings on alterations in ribonuclease (the enzymes which primarily break down the RNA that is no longer required in the cell). Ribonuclease also is involved in other important complex chemical reactions in the cell. In other words, this is part of the chemical structure of your cell that you don't want altered.

The French army contract stipulated the required study of an American agent for radiation protection labeled as W2721. It was an effective protection, but there were two serious drawbacks: First, W2721 had to be administered intravenously. Second, W2721 had to be stored at a temperature of -328°F (-200°C). These constraints, not particularly compatible with the military's needs, were without a doubt the reason why the product was later abandoned.

For biochemical reasons and because of the legendary resistance to radiation observed to occur in the *Ginkgo biloba* trees following the atomic bombings of Hiroshima and Nagasaki, Beljanski's attention focused on the leaves of the *Ginkgo* tree.

I have seen *Ginkgo biloba* trees growing in China, Japan, Europe, and in the United States. They live to be over one thousand years old. Growing to a height of 120 feet with a trunk diameter of up to four feet and believed to be living on Earth for 270 million years, the *Ginkgo biloba* tree has been cultivated throughout the world as a result of its resistance to disease. Asian cultures have applied *Ginkgo* seeds as medicinal agents for several centuries. The modern western use of *Ginkgo* has, until now, been limited exclusively to the green leaf of the tree.

Green leaf extracts of *Ginkgo biloba* are commercially available everywhere as "standard preparations." They are recommended to improve fluid circulation in the arteries, capillaries, veins or within the brain.[70] All these botanicals are prepared with various methods, but nevertheless exhibit certain contraindications. They must be applied in low dosages.

Prepared under proprietary conditions in a completely unorthodox way, and choosing material harvested at a different period in the maturation cycle of the plant, Beljanski obtained another product that he first named *Bioparyl*. This extract is made from the golden leaves of the *Ginkgo*, not the green leaves, and has been shown to play an important role in the regulation of various protein activities, in particular enzymatic proteins involved in cell mechanisms. Prepared according to the proprietary procedure developed by Beljanski, this relabeled golden-leaf *Ginkgo* extract is completely different from all other green extracts derived from the plant.

Ginkgo and Radiation Treatment

It is well-established that exposure to radiation increases reactive oxygen in the tissues, producing oxidative stress, a chemical process that disallows the body to detoxify itself and/or repair the resulting damage and free radicals formation. Free radicals are molecules in the body that are considered dangerous because they are highly chemically reactive.

At low doses, radiation may incite body burns. At higher doses, radiation may break the chemical bonds that hold the sides of the DNA ladder together as well as produce base alterations in the rungs of the DNA ladder (changing around the C,G, T, and A combinations). It can also cause the molecular strands of the DNA to break, particularly on the single separated strands of destabilized DNA, and the damage is often compounded when chemotherapy is added to the treatment.

Throughout the various chapters of this book, I have emphasized the continually increasing and additive effects of environmental pollutants on DNA. The same cumulative effect occurs with ionizing radiation and/or chemotherapy.[71] At relatively low doses of radiation, whether from the sun or cosmic rays or X-rays or microwaves, tissue burns are the first adverse side effect to occur. Medical and laboratory scientists have shown that approximately 25 percent of radiation burns induce some benign but mostly malignant tumors and that the lowered immunity resulting from such radiation and/or chemotherapy predisposes malignant degeneration.[72] It is therefore important for each individual to protect his or her skin from burns, whether from the sun or from ionizing radiation.

The golden leaf *Ginkgo biloba* plant extract prepared according to Dr. Mirko Beljanski's proprietary technique has been widely utilized in Europe for the last twenty-five years. Since the consequences of serious burns appear several months or even years later, it is interesting to evaluate the protection and satisfaction of those people who have used the *Ginkgo* extract over a length of time. Natural Source, International in conjunction with the CIRIS organization sent a questionnaire to Europeans who had undergone radiation therapy and used Beljanski's *Ginkgo biloba* to protect themselves from burns or fibrosis. Fibrosis is an abnormal amount of scar-like or fibrous tissue which may appear in skin and/or organs following injury, inflammation, burns, and radiation. Of the more than one hundred responses received and tabulated, CIRIS reports that 50 percent of the responders stated they did not experience any radiation burns, 38 percent felt the equivalent of a sunburn, and 4 percent of the patients' burns were of a more serious nature. Only one patient, who received two times the normal level of radiation, experienced a third-degree burn. This survey is highly suggestive that the golden leaf *Ginkgo* extract helps to handle, if not alleviate altogether, the burns associated with radiation. [73]

Radiation Induced Fibrosis

Radiation burns also produce fibrosis in the affected areas. The scar tissue that forms as a result of radiation exposure is insidious; it changes into diseased tissue six to twelve months after the radiation exposure.

Excessive alcohol intake can also produce fibrosis, which can lead to cirrhosis, a serious and life-threatening liver disease. In the United States each year, two-hundred thousand patients develop pulmonary fibrosis. Of these people, more than forty-thousand die annually from pneumonia, cystic fibrosis, lung fibrosis, and other associated fibrotic problems that have all been caused by persistent radiation.

How radiation toxicity may lead to fibrosis is not yet precisely known. Beljanski showed that in many cases, if not in all types of fibrosis, there are changes in nucleases, which are closely linked biochemically to collagen production. Collagen is the fibrous protein found in bone, cartilage, ligaments, skin, etc. This may explain how the *Ginkgo biloba* extract he developed diminishes scar formation, protects against fibrosis, preserves skin from undergoing the stressors of radiation burns, reduces the other numerous problems associated with chemotherapy, and neutralizes the immunological trauma connected with serious surgery. That is an impressive array of effects created by one herbal extract.

As is the case with all of Beljanski's discoveries, the science is complex but readily available to those who wish to find it in his published works. What is important to know is that Dr. Beljanski spent hundreds of hours studying ribonucleases extensively as well as the effect golden leaf *Ginkgo biloba* had on regulating cellular disruptions. [74]

The particular golden-leaf *Ginkgo biloba* extract that Dr. Beljanski developed proved to be an excellent regulator/normalizer for numerous proteins and particularly nucleases. By its regulatory and normalizing effect on cell enzymes, it enhances the natural cell repair process and helps the tissues to remain healthy, even when they are exposed to extreme physiological stressors. That is why it is so helpful for people undergoing chemotherapy and radiation. Like the RNA fragments, but working with a different mechanism, the *Ginkgo* allows radiation to do its dirty work on the cancer cells while protecting the healthy noncancerous cells. Selectivity in action, once again is exhibited, and integration with mainstream cancer therapies is obvious.

Protein Markers

By 1977, Dr. Beljanski understood that in any kind of living organism during its lifetime, little by little, the DNA accumulates substances which destabilize it. At a certain threshold of destabilization, the cellular DNA becomes deregulated, dysfunctional, and abnormal. This marks the first appearance of disease. DNA then excessively synthesizes cancer molecules—the start of cancer tumors. It is a horribly predictable cycle.

The medical community has come to rely on this cycle, however, for something called cancer "markers" to predict the onset of cancer as well as to gauge how effective (or not) their treatments are. These markers are actually proteins with names such as Prostate Specific Antigens (PSA), the marker for prostate cancer, and are generally the tell-tale signs of the start (or the abatement, if used after treatment) of cancer in a tissue, organ, or other body part.

Because protein synthesis is a vital part of the replication process, too much replication (especially that which is induced by unscheduled replication) produces too much protein. When proteins are synthesized in excess by diseased cells, they become "cancer markers." There are many different cancer or tumor markers, and they're used in oncology to help detect the presence of cancer. These markers indicate the DNA destabilization already underway. As the process continues on *ad infinitum*, it contributes to a physiological snowball effect. Dr. Beljanski was keenly aware of cancer markers and the seemingly irreversibility of the process.[75] I have no doubt the idea of "irreversibility" spurred Beljanski on to further research, and he found an answer in his golden-leafed *Ginkgo* extract.

Golden-leaf *Ginkgo* has shown itself to normalize the replication process of DNA that is marked by an excess of protein in the blood. Science has discovered protein markers for all disease; there are markers for inflammation, bone metabolism, carcinogenesis, and many more. These various proteins are very frequently generated in significant excess during the course of certain illnesses.

Bringing these protein markers back to normal values helps to restrain the progress of a disease that is underway. Through a complex process of chemical reactions on RNA and DNA, regular intake of the *Ginkgo biloba* golden leaf extract makes this normalization of proteins possible, making it, yet again, an ideal substance for integrative cancer therapies now and in the future.

While it needs more research in modern American laboratories, as of this date, Dr. Beljanski's *Ginkgo biloba* extract, like his other products, has shown no history of adverse side effects. Over time it normalizes any abnormal enzymatic activity the patient may be experiencing due to disease, toxic treatments, or radiation. It largely contributes to homeostasis by re-establishing the balance of enzymatic activity, and by facilitating the immunity through a group of specific substances.

Time for an Evolution

Those in the alternative-health community have come to distrust the products produced by Big Pharma as much as Big Pharma distrusts plant-based holistic botanicals upon which the alternative crowd relies so heavily. But with such promising results shown by the Pao pereira, *R. vomitoria*, RNA fragments, and golden-leafed *Ginkgo biloba*, is it not time to swallow our collective pride and admit that they should be included in mainstream integrative therapies?

I believe that true integration must include natural substances that are scientifically proven to be non-toxic and selective. These criteria are absolutely vital if we are truly going to find a cure for cancer that will consistently work most of the time. ("Most" because even though modern medicine now knows how to cure pneumonia, for example, it is still a deadly disease to some. Cancer, as with all disease, will always take a certain percentage of the population, no matter how effective our treatments become.)

There has been an enormous amount of research done on various cancer-fighting agents. Mirko Beljanski's decades of painstaking research gave us some of the greatest gifts to humanity: the revelation of cancerous DNA, the Oncotest, RNA-fragments along with the life-saving botanicals Pao Pereira, *R. vomitoria*, and golden-leafed *Ginkgo*. The science shows that his discoveries help alleviate the problems associated with standard cancer treatments *thereby making the standard treatments more effective.*

Before doing the research for this book, if I were to hear that dreaded sentence, "You have cancer," I would have staunchly held to the alternative treatments. Now, I wouldn't hesitate to incorporate what I know from *all* available treatments and beat the supposedly unbeatable.

Now is the time for an evolution of thought on both sides of the healing fence, establishment and holistic. Let's rise above the contention between the two camps. Lives are at stake. Our own lives as well as those we love are needlessly being lost because of a stubborn refusal to look seriously at the research already accomplished.

There is still much work to be done to show that the bolt molecules, the RNA fragments, and the specially prepared *Ginkgo biloba* extract work to enhance conventional oncological treatment.

There is no time like the present to start.

Case Study of Melanoma

"In April 2004, the tiny pimple-like bump on my thigh turned into a nightmare of distress for me. The mole-like tumor was eventually diagnosed as melanoma, a somewhat rare cancer. It required immediate removal. I was hospitalized for diagnostic testing and to ascertain my required cancer markers in order to detect whether any further tumors had developed. Even then, at sixty-two years of age, I was devastated by the thought of early death. I cried everyday as I waited for my results from the surgeon's skin biopsy." Thus began the story of French homemaker Madame Eliane Escalon (Mme. Escalon).

"The results finally came back. Yes, it was melanoma; I was nevertheless determined to put up a fight."

Melanoma is a cancer that originates in melanocytes, the pigment-producing cells of the skin. Melanocytes ordinarily give skin its distinctive color, but sunlight stimulates them to produce more melanin, the pigment that darkens the skin and increases the risk of a melanoma cancer. The lesion can begin as a new, small, pigmented skin growth on normal skin, most often on sun-exposed areas, or it may develop from preexisting pigmented moles. Sometimes melanoma runs in families. It spreads, or metastasizes, to distant parts of the body where the tumor continues to grow and destroy tissue. It's not uncommon for the melanoma lesion to appear as a firm black or gray lump as described by Mme. Escalon.[76]

Chemotherapy is used to treat melanomas that have spread, but few are cured. Some of the people treated live less than nine months; however, the course of the disease varies greatly and depends in part on the strength of the body's immune defenses. Mme. Escalon was one of the fortunate few whose immune ability was receptive to outside help, specifically to the group of correctives that had been developed by Mirko Beljanski, Ph.D. This melanoma victim went on to explain how Beljanski's products came into her possession.

"One evening, a woman in the hospital who was there as a patient asked if she could speak with me. I agreed, although I had no desire to talk about the disease that was ruining my life," continued Mme. Escalon. "Yet, it seemed as if fate had sent this person just in time to lift my spirits. The woman told me of her own mother, who also was given a death sentence by her oncologists and yet lives in full health thanks to Dr. Mirko Beljanski's herbal supplements. Beljanski was deceased by then. Having never heard of him or his plant products before, and knowing that this woman would be leaving the hospital the next day, I asked her to give me more specific information, which she did.

"Shortly thereafter, I was operated on for melanoma excision. In order to completely eradicate the approximately one-inch long tumor, the surgeon gouged a deep hole on my thigh, the circumference size of a half-grapefruit, with the expectation of performing a skin graft later on. After I was released, I contacted the Beljanski Foundation in the United States, where I received contact information for a homeopathic doctor near my home area of France. After consulting the homeopath, I ordered the supplements over the internet, and just forty-eight hours later, I was able to begin my self-treatment.

"The homeopath used my weight, 125 lbs., to figure out how many supplements to take. He prescribed nine vegetarian doses per day of the herb *Ginkgo biloba* to be swallowed over two months and then four doses of each of the other Beljanski products over ten-months' time," she told me. "Experiencing tremendous suffering from so much invasive surgery—the incision was deep and wide—I was evaluated every other day by a nurse visiting me at home with no other product for treatment except some soap and water. The visiting nurse kept my surgical wound clean and changed its dressing.

"Dr. Beljanski's supplements brought about a startling beneficial effect. My wound healed with such speed that my surgeon couldn't believe his eyes when finally I visited his office. I tried to tell the doctor that I was taking a dietary supplement for scarring, but he seemed not to care and no one in his clinic believed me. It was the nurse who had been treating me every other day, and who witnessed the favorable progress of my incision, who helped me to understand just how extraordinary—incredible even—the scar's rapid healing really was," Mme. Escalon continued. "In two months, the incision was completely closed up and I was lucky enough to learn from the doctor that a graft was no longer necessary because I had healed so quickly.

"I would like to thank Dr. Beljanski, whom I never knew, and whom the conventional medical community does not wish to recognize. Today I take his supplements as a precaution every spring and fall. Seeing how successfully my wound healed, my husband decided to take Dr. Beljanski's *Ginkgo biloba* after he underwent a bladder operation. His incision also healed up quickly. Since then, I have been a member of the CIRIS organization, and I strongly recommend Dr. Beljanski's anticancer products to anyone who will listen."

Mme. Escalon's tape-recorded testimonial is a fine example of the type of result one can expect from the use of Beljanski's herbal extracts. By taking the anticancer botanicals twice yearly, she firmly believes that she keeps the melanoma in remission. Furthermore, whatever the cause of the skin injury (incision, burn, fibrosis, radiation), the yellow leaf powder of *Ginkgo biloba* herbal medicine extract, prepared according to Dr. Beljanski's proprietary method, is of the utmost importance for health professionals to know about and for patients to use.

6

Possible Help for Those Who Suffer From HIV/AIDS

Note: While this book dedicates itself almost exclusively to reporting on Dr. Mirko Beljanski's discoveries as they relate to cancer, my publisher and I would be remiss to not inform our readers about the other significant usage of Beljanski's findings to handle HIV (Human Immunodeficiency Virus) and additional viruses, deadly or no. However, there has been almost no outside research performed on the anti-viral properties of his anticancer botanicals. Those patients infected with viral illnesses should demand more research be done based on Beljanski's research.

Until the latter part of 1985, Monsieur Gerard Weidlich, a retired French law enforcement officer, had been Chief Inspector with *Compagnie Republicaine de Securité* (CRS), the Republic of France's National Police Force. Chief Inspector Weidlich, before his retirement, trained other police officers in diving by use of Self-Contained Underwater Breathing Apparatus (SCUBA), open water rescue, water safety, and life resuscitation to save swimmers. Weidlich became famous before his retirement when he contracted AIDS in the line of duty and still lived a full life for the next twenty-four years by his self-administration of Dr. Beljanski's supplements.

Credited with personally saving the lives of over two thousand near-drowning victims, Chief Inspector Weidlich was France's life preserving troubleshooter. He regularly patrolled France's two most dangerous beaches, Canou and La Pamyre. These beaches are located along the nation's eastern and southern coasts where waves roll in sometimes at the height of three-story buildings. The currents are treacherous; the undertow, powerful. More French people drown at these two beaches than anywhere else in that nation. Those swimmers at Canou and La Pamyre beaches, indeed, seem to take excessive amounts of unnecessary risks.

It was at La Pamyre Beach on the Atlantic Ocean near the city of Bordeaux during the month of August 1985 that Weidlich contracted his infection with HIV-1. As medical consumers are now all too aware, AIDS was, at the time, uniformly lethal, most patients dying from it within two to five years.

Weidlich acquired the HIV-1 infection from administering mouth-to-mouth resuscitation in order to save the life of a near-drowned, mucous-spitting and vomiting, HIV-infected person. He took in the victim's regurgitated body fluids. Chief Inspector Weidlich absorbed HIV into his bloodstream and within a few months came down with the various illnesses related to AIDS. During the winter of 1985-86, Weidlich exhibited many of the common opportunistic infections including herpes simplex, the yeast syndrome from *Candida albicans*, fungal infections of many types, diarrhea, and severe, prolonged fatigue. At that time, the disease had only recently come upon the world scene. There was no treatment for AIDS; the generic drug azidothymidine known under its abbreviation as AZT was just about to be released.

According to the World Health Organization (WHO), since 1981 (when AIDS was first recognized as a possibly life-threatening illness), nearly thirty million people have died worldwide as of 2008. WHO also stated that in the year 2010 at least forty-two million people involving all continents became HIV-positive. They are fighting for their lives against an illness with no cure. It is a sickness that stigmatizes. Presenting a variety of signs and symptoms, the illness is surrounded by shame and mystery. Medical researchers are still debating its possible etiologies (causes) and even whether this disease is a new entity at all.

Conventional medicine treats AIDS using drug therapies that, in many instances, produce highly toxic side effects which resemble the symptoms of the illness itself. The brand-named pharmaceutical *Zidovudine*, commonly referred to as AZT, was the primary drug that mainstream medicine administered as therapy for AIDS back in 1986. It produced massive numbers of adverse post-treatment events—complications which by themselves are illnesses. After many years of treating patients with AZT, this ineffective and toxic product was taken off the market.

Shortly after Gerard Weidlich had been infected, the product was offered to him as the one-and-only-hope for AIDS patients, but he refused to take it.

With no doubt as to his AIDS diagnosis, Gerard Weidlich was allowed to leave his Chief Inspector's position at the CRS on a full disability pension. But CRS officials, feeling acute shame that one of its officers was forced to retire with a diagnosis of AIDS as his declared illness, refused to allow Chief Inspector Weidlich's real condition (his HIV infection) to be certified in the official record. Such a record usually is open to the French public. Instead, the national police force of France offered a no-hassle deal to Gerard Weidlich: "If you accept the record's statement that you retired with an injured back, we'll give you your pension starting at once and you won't need to fight us for it in court." He accepted the CRS offer, and the reason stated for his disability on his official police discharge record is, "Disability for back injury."

The life story of Monsieur Gerard Weidlich (M. Weidlich), describing how he contracted and accepted living with acquired immunodeficiency syndrome has been discussed at length in a 2003 bestselling French-language hard-cover book. Its title: *Investigation de Jean-Paul Le Perlier, Enquete Sur Un Survivant Illegal* (Jean-Paul LePerlier's Investigation of an Illegal Survivor), published by the Guy Tredaniel Editeur Publishing House.[77] As of this writing, the book is still a popular seller in many French book stores and throughout Europe.

Triumph Over AIDS

The membership organization, *Centre d'Innovations, de Recherches et d'Informations Scientifiques* (CIRIS), formed on November 24th,

1986, is comprised of mostly French people who have had their lives preserved, sometimes for many years, by following the biochemical concepts put forth by Mirko Beljanski, Ph.D. Each member had been told by an oncologist or another physician specialist that he or she was destined to die relatively soon from cancer, some other degenerative disease, or an infectious viral disease such as AIDS. CIRIS now has approximately four thousand members who are dedicated to spreading word about the discoveries developed by the microbiologist.

M. Gerard Weidlich received assistance from this same group of formerly sick people. When I met him, Gerard Weidlich had become the executive director of CIRIS. He was grateful for having Beljanski's botanicals available for the preservation of his life and elimination of symptoms. Thereafter he devoted the balance of his life to spreading word of Beljanski's discoveries throughout France and the rest of Europe.

When I interviewed him, over eighteen years after he incurred his HIV infection, Gerard remained strong, energetic, vigorous, active, and forceful. He swam in the ocean daily in the best of health, without any signs, symptoms, or complications of AIDS. I wondered how he did that so I asked, "How do you, a former policeman, achieve this remarkable result despite your starting out with blood tests recorded at an HIV positive patient stage II showing a low CD_4 to CD_8 lymphocyte blood ratio (the elements in the blood that indicate HIV infection)?"

While seated at his office desk in his well-furnished home in the South of France, Gerard explained his treatment program to me in a series of tape recordings. Monsieur Weidlich stated: "In the spring of 1986, I began a concentrated course of self-treatment with the monotherapy of a highly purified extract of Pao pereira that Dr. Mirko Beljanski provided me as a nutritional supplement in capsule form; it was then code-marked as *PB-100*.

"Dr. Beljanski had been reluctant to dispense this active ingredient because it was yet untested as a treatment for AIDS. Also, Beljanski advised that he was not a medical doctor and was not allowed to give out nutrients, even though they were not classified as drugs, since he certainly understood that they would be used by me as treatment," Gerard Weidlich said. "Yet, I desperately needed what Beljanski had discovered or invented. So I was exceedingly forceful in my arguments— I practically bludgeoned Beljanski with words into yielding on his principles. In this instance, my skills with using arguments, intimidation, pleadings, and logic on criminals came into play for persuading the microbiologist. My life was on the line, and I pulled out all the stops in my methods of persuasion.

"So I eventually acquired the Pao herbal extract from this marvelous molecular biologist," Weidlich continues. "Faithful to my regimen, I took 1 gram per day by mouth of this Pao pereira botanical. I continued following Dr. Beljanski's protocol for no less than 113 months. What happened could be considered a supernatural effect in the physical world—some might call it 'a miracle'! Being a former policeman, perhaps slightly cynical, and unquestionably a stark realist, however, I do not ever speak in terms of *miracles*. But I am alive and thriving today, so how else would you describe the effect of Beljanski's pills?

"By May 1988, testing turned up that no more HIV organisms could be found anywhere in my blood circulation. The hospital's medical doctors and laboratory technicians conducted numerous blood tests on me and each time expressed amazement at what they uncovered," he says. "My P-24 antigenemia for this disease was totally negative in June 1989."

Gerard went on to explain during our 2003 interview: "My anti-HIV antibodies became what appeared to be negative in October 1991. I was frightened because usually that's a sign of AIDS development, but then they reappeared in the beginning of September 1992 with a figure of 3125 microliters of blood, corresponding to a blood index close to a normal number of one. Let me assure you that after eighteen years of continual monotherapy using Dr. Beljanski's Pao pereira as an oral remedy,

I am in the absolute best of physical shape. I am working full time to advance the goals of CIRIS—as long as twelve hours a day."

Assisted by his wife, the occupation of Gerard Weidlich changed from being a police officer to becoming the executive director of CIRIS. He was also elected to the organization's presidency by its respectful membership who loved him. Gerard assured me during our September 2003 interview that his energy and longevity were due to his ingesting a twice daily maintenance dosage of Dr. Beljanski's Pao Pereira extract as capsules—four per day. The former Chief Inspector intended never to discontinue taking these capsules as long as he lived. Yet, he acknowledged that a relapse could strike him down at any time, even for no known reason.

At the time of our interview, Gerard Weidlich no longer had HIV circulating in his blood. While AIDS experts have told me that once the human body has contracted a virus, the viral RNA will always be present in the form of something called "proviral DNA" that is integrated into the patient's DNA blueprint. This proviral DNA can remain dormant for years, but it can be incited into activity by some anti-immunity stimulus and the pathological processes that are caused by the AIDS virus could begin once again. However, that is not what happened to Gerard Weidlich. He passed away in 2007 from a pulmonary embolism (a blockage of one of the main arteries in the lung from a clot that travelled from elsewhere in the body), the same condition that took his mother. I was notified of his death in a letter by his CIRIS staff members and was saddened to hear the news. M. Gerard Weidlich was a brave, strong man.

I have since remained in contact with members of the organization. CIRIS remains a strong organization with an expanding membership, more than half of whom have possessed various serious illnesses. It also has members who are healthy. Members of CIRIS often show a willingness to extend themselves; they make financial donations; voluntarily give up their time; offer rooms as regional meeting facilities; present verbal explanations of Dr. Beljanski's program to neighbors, friends, relatives, and meeting attendees; and engage in other constructive activities as well. These participants want to help fellow Frenchmen and others in foreign lands obtain information about how Dr. Beljanski's natural and non-toxic therapies can be useful for all people.

To acquire more information and to join forces with those who are speaking out, please contact CIRIS or The Beljanski Foundation at www.Beljanski.com or email them at info@beljanskifoundation.com. Please see Appendix A for more information.

Mirko Beljanski Becomes Involved in the Anti-Viral Fight

In 1971, a very important microbiological discovery about viruses was described by an American biochemist in the United States. Howard Temin, Ph.D., gave an account of an enzyme able to copy RNA into DNA. He is credited for discovering reverse transcriptase in viruses.[78] I described reverse transcription in chapter 5 and its importance to the HIV-infected community. However, it is from Dr. Temin's discovery that the new medical biochemical terms "reverse transcriptase" and "retrovirus" originate.

In 1972, Dr. Beljanski published another near-duplicative series of results about a bacterium rather than a virus which exhibits RNA to DNA conversion. It was an equally dramatic finding. Dr. Beljanski wrote the following new piece of information in his published article: "*In vitro* synthesis of DNA [took place] on an RNA template through an *E. coli* transcriptase."[79] He had not yet named this type of transcriptase "reverse transcriptase," but the facts are there. The following year Beljanski published two more papers on reverse transcriptase beginning with the words: "Separation from reverse transcriptase ..."[80]

Today, it is widely known that reverse transcriptase enzymes can be found in innumerable living organisms including plants, animals, bacteria, viruses, parasites, and so forth. But at the time of Temin's discovery, it was shockingly new. So new, in fact, that, even in the U.S., it took almost a year before Dr. Temin's American microbiological colleagues accepted their own colleague's findings. The professional jealousy was even worse for our French microbiologist. Despite early denials by those same semi-envious colleagues, in 1975 Howard Temin, Ph.D., and his biochemist coworker, David Baltimore, Ph.D., were awarded the Nobel Prize in Physiology or Medicine for this discovery of viral reverse transcriptase.

HIV is a retrovirus, that is to say a virus which reverses itself by having RNA transfer its genetic codes into DNA, not vice-versa. It is the actual reversed HIV-RNA microbial particle which is the infectious agent that brings on the pathological signs, symptoms, and complications of AIDS.

Biochemical scientists now know and accept as truth that viral RNA must be transcribed into DNA by reverse transcriptase in order to survive and multiply in the cell. Dr. Beljanski first observed and reported on this particular trait of certain mechanisms in bacteria. Once it was discovered that the same thing can happen in viruses, Beljanski then described the method by which his botanical discoveries worked against viral reproduction. By attaching itself to viral RNA, the alkaloid of Pao pereira blocks transcription of viral reverse transcriptase and provides the herb's effect against HIV itself. Pao pereira also blocks replication of viral DNA to regular DNA by attaching itself to the enzyme that tells the DNA to replicate: polymerase DNA. Thus, most viruses (not only HIV) are inhibited by the Pao bark extract without any toxic side effects for the infected individual. The botanical alkaloid of Pao pereira stops symptomatic actions of an RNA disease particle. (Who says the common cold can't be cured?)

These findings showing up in laboratory cultures gave Mirko Beljanski the idea to attempt to use the antiviral power of Pao pereira in plants to benefit the agricultural industry. He first chose to treat tobacco plants which are often attacked by an RNA virus called "Tobacco mosaic virus." He cured the tobacco plants of viral disease.

Then some weeks later a human Phase I pilot study was carried out to evaluate tolerance and feasibility of a twelve-month treatment in a homogeneous group of ten AIDS-related Complex (ARC) patients. This investigation was developed during the period 1990 to 1993 in the French hospital, Laperonie (a facility for people at short-term risk of full blown AIDS), and the results showed that while no drug resistance was developed, there was a tendency toward normality of all the indicators of HIV by 50 percent. [81]

The clinical study's investigators concluded that the Pao pereira extract in capsule form (code-marked PB-100 at the time, as mentioned to me by Gerard Weidlich) could be considered as a promising new drug for the effective treatment of HIV-1 infection.

Several veterinarians used the Pao extract on animals, mainly cats, which were either infected with the feline's FIV virus or with the leucosis retrovirus. It seems that the Pao extract has a very large range of possibilities against many viruses, but this work has not been sufficiently developed. It will require more animal experimenters to investigate treatment possibilities of Beljanski's products in veterinarian medicine.

Indeed, because the anecdotal evidence as well as preliminary studies are so promising, Dr. Mirko Beljanski's work is ripe ground for a thorough U.S. Government financial investment in its search for a cure of AIDS and any associated retroviruses.

AIDS specialists, alerted to a possible new therapy, have an explanation here of why within a few days of using Pao pereira extract, Gerard Weidlich's herpes infection left him, followed by the disappearance of blood-circulating HIV.

Mirko Beljanski eventually expanded his studies using the alkaloid from Pao pereira to the flu virus, plant viruses, and to the erythroblastosis virus. (Erythroblastosis is the presence of overabundant numbers of red blood cells, a condition observed in deadly anemia—known as pernicious anemia—in relapse. A virus is the underlying source of such pathology.) Potentially Beljanski held the keys for cure of these various diseases. But he did not continue with his investigations in these areas and failed to publish his results because he met with too much pharmaceutical industry opposition and all sorts of other difficulties.

Resistance arose, in part, from those promoters of conventional therapies for HIV/AIDS. The opposition came notably from those whose interest it was to promote AZT, which had just then appeared on the market, though this antiviral quickly came into question because of its irreversible side effects. As I mentioned previously, AZT was then taken off the market and replaced with anti-HIV proteases, a class of drugs which attempts to inhibit the infectious particles of HIV from maturing. These new drugs are quite popular and broadly prescribed.

Many AIDS therapists have supposed that by varying and combining several anti-HIV synthetic drugs in the form of therapeutic cocktails, the various targets of the viral proteins would be neutralized. Sometimes this combination of drug cocktails does produce some benefit for the AIDS patient, but more often such a series of cocktails merely augments the toxic effects of each of these drugs. Despite their many complicating side effects, anti-proteases are still a marked advancement over AZT. And to this day, no biological scientist has yet shown that the protease-inhibiting constituents are unusable in conjunction with Beljanski's herbal find, Pao pereira.

There is one more piece of information to know about HIV infection. Since a copy of the virus' blueprint is integrated into the invaded cell's genome, the virus can be reintroduced into the bloodstream at any time, and it is a good idea to take the Pao pereira extract continuously as a safeguard against such a potential occurrence.

All this is made possible by low to no toxicity of Pao pereira in the human system. The Amazonian rain-forest botanical is devoid of side effects as evidenced by the several thousands of patients who have taken it daily for up to twenty-five years without any apparent side effects. Moreover, as I mentioned earlier, the Pao extract is capable of crossing the blood-brain barrier, and hence it can attack viruses present in the nervous system.

The Pao extract may also fight viruses that reside in various cells, tissues, organs, and other body parts as in the thymus or lymph cells, the mucous producing cells of the pancreas, and others.

Case History of Semi-Successful AIDS Treatment

There are many instances of people infected with HIV-1 having been helped with Dr. Beljanski's products. I possess a Parisian police-department report of a situation in which an unmarried woman infected with HIV was severely addicted to street drugs. To support her need to purchase and use expensive illegal chemical substances, she performed acts of prostitution and engaged in other criminal behavior. All of her actions were performed as a means of making money. She had been arrested many times, but was let go each time without facing serious charges.

The woman, whom we'll identify by the initials MB, eventually developed full-blown AIDS but hardly responded to any conventional therapies for the condition. Doctors in the free clinics of Paris who administer different drug therapies for AIDS admitted that nothing was working for Mademoiselle MB, and anticipated that death would be coming to her soon. They made their judgments based on the woman's CD4+ blood lymphocyte counts. CD4+ blood lymphocytes determine the ability of one's immune system to protect the body from infections; counting the CD4+ is a fine measure of the severity of the damage done by HIV infection. A healthy person shows a CD4+ lymphocyte count of roughly 800 to 1,300 cells per microliter of blood.

A lymphocyte count below about 50 cells per microliter of blood is particularly dangerous because of opportunistic infections that can rapidly cause severe weight loss, blindness, or death. Any of these do commonly occur.

It was at her lowest point of health that MB learned of Beljanski's products and found some way to acquire a daily supply of his Pao pereira extract. She self-administered it for fourteen months. Her count went from 130 to 550 during that period. But then this AIDS patient was arrested, tried, and sent to prison for continuance of her prostitution. She stopped taking Beljanski's botanicals and the gains she experienced collapsed. In jail the woman underwent a resumption of the original signs and symptoms of AIDS which had brought her to death's door originally.

By sheer good luck or something else unexplainable in her destiny, she managed to survive her one-year prison sentence and came out of jail on parole after seven months. MB, finally using her common sense, didn't purchase more street drugs but rather used her meager finances to once again acquire a supply of the Pao pereira extract. She used Beljanski's products faithfully for thirteen months more when she was then lost to follow-up and has never been heard from again. [82]

Golden-leafed *Ginkgo* and Autoimmune Disorders

In chapter 5, I talk about the importance of the golden-leafed *Ginkgo* extract Dr. Beljanski found to be effective in handling the unwanted side effects of radiation treatment.

One of the less clinically studied aspects of the *Ginkgo* extract, but promising nonetheless, is its apparent ability to help those who have developed autoimmune disorders. Thanks to those observations over the years that numerous doctors shared with the Beljanski team, it is possible to confirm that for a large number of autoimmune disorders, the *Ginkgo biloba* extract, alone or in conjunction with RNA fragments (for immunity) or with the Pao pereira extract if a virus is indicated or even suspected, quite often allow for a considerable improvement in one's general condition.

Let's not forget that all of Beljanski's products are devoid of any toxic effects, are perfectly compatible with conventional treatments, and are compatible with each other in terms of supporting the immune system (often called into question with auto-immune disorders). They fight cancer cells and viruses and bring different proteins back to normal values. And in the brilliant researcher's mind, there was no doubt that, by normalizing nucleases with the botanicals, it became possible to deprive non-conforming primers of abnormal cells, cancerous, viral, or otherwise, and thus cause the cell to die for it would no longer be able to replicate.

It is only with a multi-pronged approach that a lasting improvement, even a cure, for these incapacitating diseases may be obtained. All the discoveries perfected by Mirko Beljanski, Ph.D., are mutually and synergistically beneficial as nutritional support for patients suffering from viral illnesses or various degenerative pathologies. The combination of all four major supplements Beljanski developed has proven themselves able to kill cancer cells or viral pathogens and normalize proteins. By doing this, physiological conditions for the patient are brought back to normal levels.

Used for various illnesses, the unique *Ginkgo biloba* extract proved to have regulatory functions that went far beyond what the Beljanski research team had originally hoped.

The Case of Francine Boquet

One of the most heart-warming success stories I recorded when I met with CIRIS members in 2003 was that of Madame Francine Boquet (Mme. Boquet). This homemaking wife and mother is an attractive, friendly, French matron.

With only slight embarrassment, Mme. Boquet explained her full case history to me in halting English. In 1984 at age thirty-three, Francine Boquet contracted the life-threatening HIV-1 virus that turned into full-blown AIDS. She was the unfortunate recipient of contaminated blood she received during numerous transfusions while confined to bed in a Parisian hospital. This situation occurred after she hemorrhaged following surgery for a hysterectomy. At least some of this blood obtained from the French National Blood Bank was contaminated with the HIV virus and these viruses invaded her tissues.

Madame Francine Boquet's Interview

"Yes, yes, yes! I give permission for you to publish my story and print my photograph," stated Francine Boquet emphatically when I asked her if I could.

"You see, I suffered a severe hemorrhage in 1984 from undergoing a total hysterectomy and sixty-nine bags of blood given to me during that time were needed to save my life.

"Perhaps the blood did save me, but a month later the first in a series of disabling symptoms and signs began that would last for the next four years. The transfused blood had been contaminated, the hospital later admitted.

"Because of my profuse gynecological bleeding, I had been forced to receive a lot of blood, and all of it was bad. *(Author's note: While it is doubtful that all of the blood was bad, just a few contaminated units could have made Mme. Boquet HIV positive.)* Of course, I did not know about the blood transfusion impurities—not even for four years afterward. I never had any suspicions. Until the transfusions occurred, I had been a healthy and happy woman, very active, dynamic, a work producer, caretaker of my children, an efficient housekeeper, and a responsive wife," continues Mme Boquet. "Afterward I went through absolute hell from my many illnesses. I suffered as a mother, in my marriage, socially, as a housewife, at my part-time job that I had to leave—I suffered in all ways!

"Following my receiving the contaminated blood, from 1984 to 1988, I experienced severe diarrhea, weight loss, urinary tract problems, and felt just plain dirty inside and out. Also I felt awash with constant fatigue—tired, worn out, fully exhausted even when getting up in the morning—a very difficult situation that devastates me even now as I think of it twenty years later," the homemaker remembered as tears rolled down her cheeks. "I want to talk about my problems today in order to help others by supplying them with useful information that I have learned the hard way.

"By 1988, Parisians had begun to talk about HIV infection as the cause of this very deadly disease referred to as AIDS. At first I believed that HIV and AIDS had nothing to do with me, but chronic fatigue syndrome was part of the symptoms that people were discussing, and I felt devastating fatigue all of the time. It wasn't until my mother arrived for an extended visit with my family that I consulted a homeopathic physician about the fatigue. My mother pushed me to get a medical checkup. The doctor performed all kinds of examinations on me including blood tests. He immediately suspected HIV and during the first visit, he warned me, saying 'You are a potential HIV candidate patient.'

"But this was a relatively new disease, and the homeopath's diagnosis was not made definitive until seven days later. I kept the bad news from my husband until after the second visit to my doctor, for I did not know how Alain would react to it.

"So at my return visit, I received the full results of the doctor's tests, including information about the infectious organisms in my blood. I learned that I was infected with both hepatitis C and HIV. My understanding was that this was my death sentence. I kept saying over and over: 'It's not fair, it's not fair! What did I do to deserve this?'

"The doctor told me, 'Having been infected in this way for four years, it's a miracle you are still alive.' It was then that I lost my voice—probably from shock. I went home speechless and in a daze," Mme. Boquet affirms. "The worst-case scenario that went through my mind was that I may have given the infection to Alain. My two small children could lose both of their parents. My whole life seemed to have fallen apart. Yet, it was my duty to tell my husband, and I did.

"Alain took me to a specialist in AIDS care who offered me conventional medical treatment for my problem—AZT. I categorically refused the drug because of how the medical establishment had abused me with its careless methods of blood management and the resultant contamination. I declared that even if my 1984 operation had saved my life, the transfusions had taken it away again. When I verbalized my strong opinion and refused the standard AIDS treatment, this specialist surprised me by not arguing but rather offering me an alternative method of healing," says Mme Boquet. "The physician referred me to two other French patients infected with full blown AIDS, Gerard Weidlich and a handsome young man named Mark Schreiber. I learned that the two patients were remaining comfortable and symptom-free as a result of their taking certain treatments developed by a biochemist named Dr. Mirko Beljanski.

"My AIDS specialist, an M.D., had read published scientific articles by Dr. Beljanski; he had met these two patients who confirmed that Beljanski's literature was valid. Much later I met the same two men and had my picture taken with them. So, while he did not necessarily advise me to take them, the AIDS specialist told me of the existence of plant products developed by Dr. Beljanski," the woman states. "Then he proceeded to find out how I might acquire them for personal use. I waited only a short time for his information. The physician telephoned back within twenty-four hours with the name, address, and phone number of Dr. Beljanski so that Alain and I went right away to meet with the scientist in his modest research laboratory in a townhouse located on the outskirts of Paris.

"Having spent at least ninety minutes with Beljanski, we felt quite at ease with this scholarly, gentle man. It was my sense that positive things could happen for me by using his nutritional molecules. He did say to us, 'I am not a medical doctor but rather a biochemist and can't guarantee anything. Also, my advice is that you have a number of additional laboratory tests performed by your physician.' So I did what he asked," Mme Boquet responded. "The tests were performed, results supplied to us, and Dr. Beljanski provided me with Pao pereira and *Ginkgo biloba*. I began taking both of these herbs as capsules at once, two of each, three times daily, amounting to twelve pills at a dosage of four in the morning, four in the afternoon, and four at night."

The Pao botanical extract Mme. Boquet took was the same concoction cancer victims take. The *Ginkgo biloba* extract was meant to help with Mme. Boquet's enzymes, especially her transaminases, which were deregulated by the virus. Transaminases are enzymes that when elevated indicate liver damage.

"Dr. Beljanski's conscientiousness and his attention to my need for help inspired confidence in Alain and me. I followed his directions to the letter, and after a month I felt so much better—diarrhea stopped and much less fatigue was present. I could take care of my children and do my housework once again," adds Francine Boquet. "I took Beljanski's botanicals regularly over the course of many months when I realized, subtly and for the first time in years, that my cystitis and other urinary tract infections had disappeared. Since the day I started taking Dr. Beljanski's products, I have not gotten sick again. I became much more energetic and could accomplish my daily chores.

"At first my husband refused to be tested for AIDS to avoid insulting or embarrassing me, but Dr. Beljanski insisted on such testing in his very dynamic manner. Alain finally did get the HIV blood test, and it turned out to be negative," states Mme Boquet. "As my health improved steadily, my husband became more and more grateful. Thus, he eventually volunteered two full days a week in the Beljanski laboratory just to help out as an assistant.

"For me it was a wonderful thing that I could have found Dr. Mirko Beljanski; quite simply his botanicals are responsible for eliminating the signs, symptoms, and complications of AIDS from ruining the lives of my family and me. Out of thousands of French people who died from transfused blood contaminated with HIV in 1984, I am among those very few remaining alive whose survival comes directly from this microbiologist's laboratory workbench," Mme. Boquet stated emphatically. "I continue to take my capsules every day and will do so as long as I live."

Thirty months after our above-reported interview with Mme. Francine Boquet, the woman advised me that she continued to feel in the best of health with no signs or symptoms of AIDS, and it had been twenty-two years since she had first contracted the disease.

Mme. Francine Boquet had been infected with one of the two labeled viruses, HIV-1 and HIV-2, that progressively destroys human white blood cells. Note that HIV-2 is seen mostly in West Africans. Infection with the HIV-1 organism observed most frequently in Europeans and North Americans brings on the indications of AIDS plus other opportunistic diseases that result from an impaired immunity. Mme. Boquet, consequently, was additionally a victim of the opportunistic illness, hepatitis C. This type of hepatitis is the most common form of post-transfusion blood infection resulting in asymptomatic chronic liver disease, including cirrhosis. From ingesting Dr. Beljanski's botanicals, however, when the woman got rid of the several symptomatic illnesses related to AIDS, her hepatitis condition disappeared as well. Thanks to Beljanski's research on viral RNA, Mme. Boquet can lead a normal life and continues to do so as of the publication of this book.

More Research to be Done

Just as more research needs to be done on Beljanski's discoveries and their effects on cancer both by themselves and coupled with conventional cancer treatments, so too does the promising effects of the Pao pereira and the *Ginkgo biloba* on HIV and other deadly viruses. These extracts need to be studied *in vitro*, *in vivo*, and in clinical trials. Yes, studies like these are costly, but there is already an enormous amount of money being spent on viral diseases.

In 2009, the latest year for AIDS statistics I was able to acquire, an estimated thirty-three million people had AIDS with 1.8 million people dying from the disease. Cancer claims about seven and a half million people a year, and while cancer is far more deadly, AIDS is just as frightening a disease. According to conventional wisdom, it resists a cure. According to some sources, no less than $7.7 billion was spent on the experiments for AIDS in 2009, including research and treatment.[83] As a comparison, the National Cancer Institute reported that $4.6 billion was spent annually on cancer research alone in 2009. [84]

Doesn't it make sense to spend some of that money on substances that have already shown themselves to be effective against cancer and AIDs jointly, both clinically and anecdotally as evidenced by the thousands of people who have used them for purposes of living normal lives?

Don't we all, especially those we love who suffer, deserve that?

7

Cancer Prevention

U p to this point, I have discussed the early detection and possible cure of life-threatening illness through applications of microbiological discoveries directly related to the living cell. But this presentation on cancer's causes and possible cures would be flawed if I did not address one of the most important aspects of any illness and its source of pathology: *prevention*. Prevention of cancer, as with any illness deadly or not, has even greater significance than its treatment, for if you can prevent something from happening in the first place, you're well ahead of the game.

When living cells malfunction, disease begins to manifest itself in the body's tissues, organs, and/or other body parts. A state of healing becomes mandatory. Your body reacts and often is capable of healing itself unless the malfunctions overwhelm what the body can physically accomplish. If the immune system is weak, the body cannot fight infection. If a tissue is over-exposed to poisons or environmental toxins, too many cells suffer from DNA destabilization; the cells replicate out of control and cancer results.

Prevention is really nothing more than strengthening one's body and mind so that its own natural defenses can work to heal. And while the possibilities of integrative treatments for those who already have cancer are promising, self-application of Dr. Mirko Beljanski's botanicals may be most effective in the area of prevention.

However, no method of disease prevention contains a magic bullet. You cannot just take a pill and believe all is well, that you'll never get sick. It takes a more concerted effort at staying healthy, and you'll need to follow a series of prevention steps to achieve total health.

Prevention Step One: Avoidance

If cancer is caused by carcinogens, and carcinogens are made up of environmental toxins and poisons, it makes logical sense that we must avoid those environmental carcinogens as much as we possibly can. In chapter 3, I offered you a very brief list of known carcinogens. There are thousands more, but instead of getting overwhelmed about their avoidance, just be smart about your personal prevention procedures. The following address what I believe to be the most important impediments against illness. I am sure there are more, but one must start somewhere:

Food

Carcinogens generally are man-made, which means that they are chemicals. If you've ever looked at the ingredients on a bag of Cheetos, Twinkies, or any other kind of junk food, you know that it's made up of a laundry list of unpronounceable chemicals. Those dyes and food additives on the label are non-nutrients and, while they have been deemed "safe" by the Food and Drug Administration, they may not be safe at all. Realize that a lot of politicking goes on behind the scenes at the Food and Drug Administration. Until Dr. Mirko Beljanski's Oncotest becomes mainstream, and thus an easy and inexpensive way to test for carcinogens is available to us, it is much better to avoid the ingestion of all those chemicals. How do you do that? Read those labels. Get educated and keep your consumption of processed food (food that has chemical additives—preservatives, binders, color enhancers, flavor enhancers, stabilizers, emulsifiers, etc.) to a minimum or avoid them altogether.

There is nothing wrong with eating meat, but meat that has been filled with growth hormones is something to avoid. I recommend eating meat that is either organic or labeled "natural" which means that a farmer's cows, pigs, and poultry are not fed antibiotics or hormones, and their meats are unprocessed (unlike hot dogs) with preservatives. It's illegal to feed poultry growth hormones in the U.S., but organic chicken is far better for you because it's not laden with antibiotics—and it tastes better too!

The growth hormone rBGH in milk has been shown to cause cancer. Knowing what we do about excessive hormones and DNA destabilization, it makes sense to avoid rBGH in all your dairy, including cheese. Buy dairy foods that do not have rBGH.

I would also tell you to eat more vegetables and fruit, but even then not all veggies are safe. Veggies you buy at the corner market, unless they are labeled organic, have residual pesticides on them and many have been irradiated. We're exposed to enough radiation through medical X-rays and such. Why expose our bodies to more radiation in our food? Buy organic! And if you think that organic is more expensive, you're correct. Still, think about how much it costs if you get cancer. Some rounds of conventional cancer treatment reach prices beyond $100,000 or more, and costs are rising 15 percent a year. [85] So you may spend more money at the grocery store buying organic food, but taking this preventative step could save you thousands of dollars and an enormous amount of grief.

Here is a final point on food and beverages which I can't stress enough. *Drink purified water only*—reverse osmosis or filtered or distilled. Chemicals in water, primarily the chlorine that is inserted to kill germs, are highly toxic. Some effective but inexpensive filters are being marketed. You can also spend a small fortune buying bottled water, but recent studies have come out suggesting that the plastic polymers in the water storage bottles leach into their contents if the water gets hot. Plastic polymers can be carcinogenic. You also don't know if that bottle you're drinking from has been sitting on the importation dock somewhere getting warm. So use caution when buying bottled water (which dollar for dollar is sometimes more expensive than gasoline). Some plastics are safer than others and a quick Google search will inform you of which are safe and which you should avoid.

The Cancer Prevention Diet

If you should avoid certain foods to prevent cancer, then that naturally begs the question: what *should* you eat?

The most favorable cancer-prevention eating plan I have ever uncovered is one developed by urologist Ronald E. Wheeler, M.D., of Sarasota, Florida, which furnishes you with a daily program of eating what he calls Modified Mediterranean Cuisine. I have modified it some, but the benefit of eating according to Wheeler's guidelines includes the maintenance of heart health plus the prevention of all cancers, but it is especially effective for prostate homeostasis (Dr. Wheeler specializes in prostate health). It also has the added plus that it may slow the aging process. Always remember that you should consult a physician or other medical practitioner before embarking on any major dietary change, and, most important, what follows are guidelines, not absolutes.

Dr. Wheeler divides his dietary plan into categories which begin with eating many kinds of fresh fruits. Here it is:

Fresh Fruits

The list Dr. Wheeler recommends includes but is not limited to:

oranges, tangerines, bananas, cherries, grapefruit, watermelon, cantaloupe, guava, kiwi, strawberries, blueberries, raspberries, blackberries, cranberries, papaya, grapes, apples, pomegranate, plums, etcetera. *Minimal to moderate intake of fruit juice.*

Fresh Vegetables

Eat fresh, never canned vegetables with the exception of tomato paste and stewed tomatoes. Examples include but are not limited to vegetables in the cabbage family including broccoli, broccolini, brussel sprouts, kohlrabi, kale, collard greens, bok choy, mustard greens, cabbage, and cauliflower. Other good vegetables to eat include but are not limited to tomatoes and tomato-related products including the aforementioned tomato paste, stewed tomatoes and tomato sauce; peppers including chili pepper, bell pepper, habanera pepper etc.; onions, peas, carrots, spinach, beets, string beans, mushrooms (shitake, portabella, morel, maitake, oyster, porcini etc.). Steamed, sautéed or wok-prepared vegetables are most nutritious. *Limit corn and corn-related products and recipes* (corn is one of the more highly-allergenic foods). Avoid fried onion rings.

Cooking Oils

Olive oil is best; peanut, sesame, sunflower, safflower, pumpkin-seed, krill (from the food whales eat) are all viable alternatives when olive oil can't be used. *Avoid palm oil, coconut oil, corn oil, and vegetable oil.*

Garnish

Garnish and/or integrate any dish with garlic, cucumbers, lettuce, celery, cumin, cilantro, pepper, oregano, ginger, rosemary, thyme, parsley, sage, mustard, relish pickles, olives, pimento, etcetera. *Avoid the use of mayonnaise and creamy bread spreads.*

Protein Sources

Cold-water fish including but not limited to tuna fresh or canned (in water or olive oil), wild salmon whenever possible, halibut, sardines, and mackerel.

Poultry including turkey and chicken (white meat only, without skin), turkey bacon, turkey sausage.

Shell fish including scallops, shrimp, crab, lobster and calamari are okay depending on the preparation.

Other forms: beans (all types), egg whites and peanut butter.

Avoid egg yolks. Limit red meat intake and make sure it is hormone and antibiotic free; organic meat is best because the feed does not include pesticides and herbicides as well. Meat to avoid: anything that is smoked or cured such as hot dogs, sausage, kielbasa, prosciutto, pepperoni, salami, bologna, Lebanon bologna, head cheese, organ meats, spam, or ham; also it is wise to avoid pork altogether (bacon and pork roll included) as well as lamb and wild game. Fish to avoid: tile fish (Tilapia), sword fish and farm-raised salmon.

Dr. Wheeler also recommends you do not eat hamburger, chili with ground beef, barbecued beef, steaks, prime rib, chicken wings, or sloppy joes.

Dairy

Eat non-fat yogurt, egg whites or egg beaters, skim milk, non-fat cheese, non-fat cottage cheese, etcetera. *Avoid fat associated with dairy including cheese, whole milk, half & half, cream, ice cream, and cream sauces including but not limited to hollandaise, béarnaise and giblet gravy.*

Pasta and/or Carbohydrates

Complex pasta made with spinach, whole-wheat, rice, brown rice or any whole-grain alternative wheat such as spelt or kamut are best. Whole-grain breads are encouraged. Moderate consumption of pizza with whole wheat crust is best. Sweet potatoes are preferred over white baking potatoes although the skins of both are nutritious. *Limit simple pasta like spaghetti and noodles while avoiding bread sticks, white bread, white rice and simple sugars such as refined white sugar and honey; avoid French-fried potatoes unless they are cut thin and fried in olive oil.*

There are many good refined sugar substitutes on the market. They include Stevia (it is now available in a non-bitter formula) and Xylitol. Both can be used for cooking and as an additive. You can also use honey, agave, maple syrup, brown rice syrup, barley malt, even molasses if you don't mind the aftertaste, but these are not sugar substitutes, just acceptable alternative forms of sugar.

Salads

Prepare fresh garden greens with cucumbers, tomatoes, avocado, raisins, radishes, onions, peppers, olives, carrots, nuts and fresh vegetables to suit. Minimally eat one salad daily. The best salad dressing is extra virgin olive oil and balsamic vinegar or red-wine vinegar (or squeeze the juice of half a lemon for a nice alternative). *Salad dressings to avoid include thousand island, creamy Italian, creamy garlic, creamy anything, French, blue cheese, and ranch. Avoid croutons.*

Whole Grains

Eat granola (homemade), oatmeal, Grape Nuts, rye, wheat, and sesame, and of course brown rice. Alternative grains such as millet, kamut, or spelt are good. *Surprisingly, Dr. Wheeler advises to avoid Flax whenever possible.*

Crackers

Any whole grain cracker is best. *Avoid crackers made with partially hydrogenated oils including but not limited to cottonseed oil and soy bean oil* (they contain trans-fats).

Soups

Eat tomato with vegetables, tomato alone, chicken with rice, chicken noodle, anything with vegetables and poultry. *Avoid cream-based soups.*

Desserts

Eat seasonal berries or a piece of dark chocolate (if you must). *Avoid pastries, cheese cake, cookies, cake, ice cream, and pies.*

Soy

Use only a moderate amount of soy including Genistein and Diadzein components. Additional soy that may be consumed but is not necessarily recommended include: soy milk, soy cheese, soy nuts, soy beans, miso, tofu, and tempeh. *Avoid Soy Sauce based on its high salt content.*

Snack Foods (in moderation)

Eat pretzels (non-fat), peanuts, hazelnuts, pistachios, Brazil nuts, almonds, walnuts, pecans, filberts, grapes, dark chocolate, trail mix (homemade), dried fruits, air-popped popcorn, matzos, a piece of fresh fruit. *Avoid soft drinks, potato chips, corn chips, candy, milk chocolate, pork rinds, microwave popcorn, cookies, Goldfish, cheese twists, etcetera.*

Beverages

Drink reverse-osmosis water (for a nice twist squeeze a lemon or lime wedge in the water); it is best to drink three to four, six- to eight-ounce glasses per day; green and red teas with a wedge of lemon squeezed into the tea prior to consumption; concord grape juice; red wine as an evening beverage (one to two 6 oz. glasses is recommended) daily; moderate the intake of any alcoholic beverage including vodka, whiskey, tequila, gin, scotch, rum, beer, assorted after-dinner drinks, and wine. *Avoid: milk shakes, soft drinks, cream liquors, schnapps, or any high-sugar liqueur.*

Supplemental Nutrition

Any valid nutrient formulation that has been proven to be beneficial is part of any good diet. Vitamins that are food based are far superior to vitamins that have been manufactured synthetically. Also it has been found that omega 3 fatty acids including 1600 mg of Eicosapentaenoic Acid (EPA) and 800 mg of Docosahexaenoic Acid (DHA) ingested daily can help decrease cancer cell proliferation and balance lipids including LDL/HDL, total cholesterol/HDL, EPA/Arachidonic Acid Ratios, and Quercetin for pelvic pain syndrome.

Supplemental nutrition specifically for prostate impairments: Supplementation can be very effective, but it best to check with your doctor or nutritionist on what works best for you, your body, and whatever ailment you're wanting to correct.

General Dietary Considerations

- Avoid fried foods whenever possible in favor of broiled or baked.
- If dieting, precede every meal with an eight-ounce glass of water.
- Heart health and cancer prevention are directly related to a proper diet.
- Get appropriate nutrition, adequate exercise, and rest.
- Practice stress reduction and get educated about an optimal lifestyle.
- Always eat food fresh and/or fresh frozen; canned goods are generally to be avoided due to preservatives.
- If you grill your dinner, do not overcook or burn what is to be consumed.
- Avoid the use of butter or margarine remembering, "If it is solid at room temperature, you shouldn't use it" (referring to butter or butter-like spreads).
- 15 percent of your daily calories should come from fats.

(NOTE: This dietary eating plan was edited by Dr. Ronald Wheeler for use by prostate-impaired patients and all other medical consumers, both women and men, on February 6, 2006.)

Household Chemicals

The liquids and powders we use to clean our houses, unless they are made from nature, are a shoo-in for being carcinogenic. Sure, they get your house shiny clean, but is it worth breathing in all those nasty chemical poisons or soaking them into one's body through the skin? Look at a bottle of your average household cleanser next time you're in the store and be prepared for label shock. Again, until the Oncotest becomes used in all research by our government and private industry to find out what is safe and what isn't, better to err on the side of being safe.

Use vinegar and water to clean; when heated together they make a marvelous disinfectant. For example, anyone with hard wood floors should know how nice such floors can look with a quick mopping of a vinegar-and-water solution. Or try a non-petroleum-based dishwashing liquid. It doesn't contain harsh chemicals that are more likely to be carcinogenic, and it cleans just as good as the other stuff. There are also a number of quality cleaning products out there made from all natural ingredients which are quite adequate cleaners and don't cost a whole lot more than the chemically-laden products. Again, think of your health when you're buying cleaning products and you may save thousands down the line.

Industrial Chemicals

People who perform blue-collar jobs tend to work around highly carcinogenic chemicals. But if your building has just been remodeled, the chemicals in the paint and the carpet can be highly toxic. If you work in a highly toxic environment, there are natural products—essential oils for example—that can help neutralize the poisons. Also, a double dose of minerals can help leach out the chemicals from your system. (Always make sure you have the proper mineral balances and combinations such as calcium with magnesium and zinc with copper. If you're ingesting salt for flavor, always take potassium to neutralize the sodium. Check with a naturopath or other qualified health professional for proper dosages of each mineral.)

Get Smart

Because there are so many, it is impossible to address all of the various classes of chemicals that can cause DNA destabilization and lead to cancer. The trick is to get smart about what are known carcinogens and what are potential carcinogens and to use that information wisely.

Please do make the effort to get some good cardio-vascular exercise in at least three times a week. The benefits of exercise are well known, but like anything else that's "good for you," it takes discipline and will power to keep up a good program. It really doesn't matter what you choose to do: walk, run, bike, rake your lawn, play a game of basketball, whatever gets your heart beat up, do it. Exercise will help you feel better and chances are, it will enhance your body's immune system, and that's always a good thing. Right?

Prevention Step Two: Detoxification

I can't stress this point enough. Detoxifying your body on a regular basis is, perhaps, the most important cancer-prevention step you can take. It is virtually impossible to keep yourself safe from all carcinogenic toxins and poisons in our modern world. If you live in a city, you're bombarded with thousands of toxins from car exhaust, chimney smoke, pesticides and herbicides we dump by the ton on our lawns. They keep the lawn green but at what cost to health? If you live in the country and close to farming areas, chances are your air is periodically polluted with pesticides and herbicides.

Fortunately our bodies are hardwired in such a way that they detoxify down to the cellular level. Our job is to help our body do its tasks in the most efficient way possible, and we can do that by taking the time and making the effort to go through various self-cleanses of sorts.

There are very many effective ways to clean out the tissues, organs, and other body parts, especially the internal organs charged with eliminating external poisons, namely the liver, kidneys, the small and large intestines, spleen, the lungs, and the gall bladder. Natural products are available to help you to purify your colon. Detoxifying is not necessarily a pleasant experience, but you will feel marvelous after doing so. Liver cleanses are simple—drinking some sort of monounsaturated oil such as olive oil with lemon juice works quite nicely.

The Gerson Therapy is a procedure I use regularly—perhaps for two days every couple of months. Dr. Gerson recommends imbibing in large amounts (thirteen eight-ounce glasses daily) of carrot juice and green juices from blended vegetables, plus the self-administration of coffee enemas. (See Appendix A for more information.)

Here are instructions from Max Gerson, M.D. on how to take a coffee enema:

> To make enemas most effective, the patient should lie on his right side, with both legs drawn close to the abdomen, and breathe deeply, in order to suck the greatest amount of fluid into all parts of the colon. The enema's fluid should be retained ten to fifteen minutes. Within twelve minutes nearly all the caffeine from organic coffee is absorbed through the bowel wall into the hemorrhoidal veins and then from these blood vessels it flows directly into the portal veins and then into the liver. Fluid expulsion offers you the feeling of complete cleanliness and good health.

For the best coffee enema concentration, do the following:

1. Drop three rounded tablespoonful's of organic ground (drip) coffee (never instant) into one quart of distilled water. (The organic coffee won't contain any adverse additives.)
2. Let the solution boil three minutes in your coffee maker and then simmer fifteen minutes more.
3. Strain the solution though a fine-mesh filter.
4. Fill a quart glass container with the liquid and let cool to body temperature.
5. Use this solution at body temperature for purposes of bowel infusion by application of an enema bucket or bag raised just eighteen inches above the anus.
6. Use a timer for the ten to fifteen minutes you are allowing the coffee to do its cleansing internally.

There's much more to detoxification than just taking an enema using organic coffee. Visit your local health-food store and ask about the various cleanses available to you. Try one. If it doesn't make you feel noticeably better, don't worry. You haven't wasted your money. You probably just need to detox more often. Whatever you do to detoxify your body will help get rid of those nasty, DNA-destabilizing poisons and toxins from your body. Detoxifying is not necessarily easy to do, and a good cleanse takes discipline. But again, isn't it better to go through a little discomfort every once in a while, but feel great afterwards, than have to go through the debilitating side effects of conventional cancer treatments?

Chelation Therapy

Chelation therapy is the process of removing heavy metal from the blood stream by various means. *EDTA* (EthyleneDiamineTetraacetic Acid) *chelation therapy* is the best physiological detoxifier of heavy metals and other metallic ions known to humans. It's administered in three ways: intravenously, orally, or anally. All administrative techniques have been found to be safe, effective, and relatively inexpensive for purposes of removing toxic metals from all parts of the body and restoring blood flow in victims of atherosclerosis. I believe strongly in the efficacy of this treatment.

During the **intravenous (IV) chelation process,** the ions of minerals floating in your bloodstream or other tissue fluids are captured and bonded into ringed structures by a chemical agent, usually a synthetic amino acid or weak organic acid that you take into your systemic circulation. The ions and the agent eventually leave your body through its usual waste disposal system. It is an arterial cleaning process. Strictly for purposes of detoxification of impurities from my body, I have received 566 intravenous chelations to date and anticipate taking more. The protocol followed by my chelating physician for intravenous chelation administration is one that's recommended by ACAM, the American College for Advancement in Medicine.

Oral chelation therapy actually is merely a term of reference, long-time used and somewhat misnamed, indicating that certain nutrients taken by mouth are acting as cellular detoxifiers. They tend to clean out waste products, pollutants, heavy metals, foreign proteins, and other toxic substances in the cells, or by diluting the electromagnetic energy stored in destructive free radicals which have been created by combining reactions within the tissues. The so-called oral-chelating agents may include anti-oxidant nutrients, pharmaceuticals, metabolic factors, food substances, dietary supplements, herbs, homeopathic botanicals, nutritional formulations, and other such ingredients, as well as specific exercises promoting a person's own systemic chelation.

Anal chelation therapy is the application of a time release suppository into the rectum just before going to sleep for the night. It is comprised of several ingredients including cocoa butter, methocel E4M premium USP, but especially the active detoxifying agent of 750 mg of calcium disodium EDTA.

For a physician near to your location, please see the membership list provided on the ACAM's website (American College for Advancement in Medicine): http://www.acamnet.org. Please also see Appendix A for more information.)

Prevention Step Three: Using Botanicals for Healing

Prevention, looked at from an alternative view, also incorporates another aspect of self-healing. The body is often in a weakened state long before manifestations of disease, and one of the most effective cancer prevention strategies is to handle the earliest indication before it gets out of hand. Those in the alternative-health community, often referred to as CAIM (Complementary, Alternative, and Integrative Medicine), know that sometimes giving the body a boost with herbal botanicals is exactly what is needed to handle a low-level infection. This way the body can get back to its normal state of health and healing.

Healing has its roots in the Greek word *holos*, from the same derivation that has given us "whole" and "holistic". Over multiple centuries, healing has developed its own descriptive language such as "life-force" (English), "*Qi*" (Chinese), "*Prana*" (Indian), "*Ki*" (Japanese), "chakras" (Indian), "emotions," "spiritual flow," "mental images," and more. These terms are as important to health as is the state of organs and tissues within the physical body. Whether we are concerned about remaining healthy, regaining health, or moving to greater health, the whole of the being, physical, mental and spiritual, is involved in the process. [86]

One hundred and fifty or so years ago, before the advent of our overly commercialized pharmaceutical industry and before the outgrowth of modern medical practitioners, Western medicine was not administered by medical doctors. Rather healing botanicals derived from nature were given out by homeopaths and naturopaths. Such naturalists were holistic in their healing techniques and utilized very few drugs, sometimes none at all. Instead, these homeopaths or naturopaths or herbalists were practitioners of botanical medicine who recognized that plant botanicals work on the whole person, not just on specific systems as do drugs or mechanical devices. Herbal medicine recognizes that botanical agents work synergistically to bring about a vastly greater effect than their individual constituents.

Two experts on natural medicine, both faculty members at the Bastyr College of Naturopathic Medicine in Washington State, tend to agree with me and countless others on this topic. In their own published book, *Encyclopedia of Natural Medicine*, a classic in its field, Michael Murray, N.D., and Joseph Pizzorno, N.D., emphasize the healing power of nature or *Vis medicatrix naturae*—. The two naturopaths state that fundamental to the practice of naturopathic medicine is a profound belief in the ability of the body to heal itself, given the proper opportunity. "The strict corollary of this is, to quote Hippocrates, 'do no evil,' *i.e.* to very carefully avoid both practices which weaken the body's ability to heal itself and therapies which take over a function of the body [the usual procedure in modern medicine]. Needless to say, this philosophy [of do no evil] has limits, and at times the body needs more than just supportive help. . . . Plants have been used as medicines since antiquity."[87]

Botanical Applications for the Elimination of Illnesses

The folklorian, superstitious, cultural, or religious use of plants and plant substances by humankind for the elimination of illnesses most likely has existed since the dawn of time, but the scientific investigation of herbal botanicals, labeled as *herbalism* or *herbology*, is a relatively recent development.

Herbs are the primary healing tools of naturopathic physicians. A Doctor of Naturopathy [N.D.] graduates after four years of undergraduate college and another four years of health care training in herbology, natural food diets, light therapy, hyperthermia, massage, fresh air inhalation, aromatherapy, homeopathy, exercise training, and the avoidance of drugs. An American N.D. practices under the code of healing which teaches that illness can be eliminated by the application of natural and non-toxic treatments. It's readily seen that treatment with herbology is the most natural healing science available anywhere.

The term *herb* here refers to a plant used for medicinal purposes and does not include the recent fad of employing "medical marijuana." Osteopaths, medical doctors, and pharmacists trained in the United States are usually incorrectly taught that the use of herbs is merely a reflection of folklore, outdated theories, and myth. In part that is because the pharmaceutical industry makes its money by manufacturing, patenting, and selling *synthetic* drugs. Their ideas have come to dominate the current culture of healing and tend to dictate how medicine should be practiced in the United States, Canada, and other western nations. No matter what you think about the pharmaceutical industry, it is a certainty that ill Americans receive drugs and hardly ever have exposure to herbs. It is also a sad but true fact that herbal therapy competes too much with drug sales, so some in the pharmaceutical industry pay multimillions of dollars to support false propaganda about herbal treatment.

There is no escaping the pharmaceutical industry's all-pervasive propaganda against herbal botanicals. Herbal botanicals are almost never mentioned in the mainstream, yet in 2007, the date of the last study done on this matter, consumers spent a reported $15 billion just on nutritional supplements such as vitamins and minerals taken as tablets, liquids and capsules plus a total of $34 billion on alternative health care, including chiropractic and acupuncture.[88] By now, with the public's new enlightenment in 2011 and its movement toward green medicine, those figures are likely to have tripled.

The situation regarding herbal medicine in the United States is considerably different in other countries except France, which is even more limiting than the U.S. in terms of governmental restrictions. Most nations around the world have numerous medical doctors and clinics practicing herbology and also homeopathy.

Germany's herbal therapies match the number of drug prescriptions written in that country. This is an astounding statistic, and it is because in that European country herbal products are marketed with drug claims if they have been proven to be safe and effective. The legal requirements for herbal medicines are identical to those of all other drugs. Herbal products sold in Germany's pharmacies are reimbursed by health insurance if they are prescribed by a physician.[89]

The proof required by a manufacturer in Germany to illustrate safety and effectiveness for the herbal product is far less than the proof required by the U.S. Food & Drug Administration for any pharmaceutical in the United States. In Germany, a special commission known as *Commission E* developed a series of two hundred monographs on herbal products similar to the over-the-counter monographs in the U.S.[90] An herbal product is viewed as safe and effective if a manufacturer meets the quality requirements of the monograph or produces additional evidence of safety and effectiveness that can include data from existing literature, anecdotal information from practicing physicians, as well as limited clinical studies.

In Asia, Central America, and South America, herbs are highly respected for healing of all sorts. I have visited hospitals in Shanghai, Beijing, and Nanking, China, and viewed entire departments administering treatment which took up several hospital floors for the preparation of herbal medicines. In the International Hospital of Beijing, I saw over six thousand drawers packed with botanicals and other ingredients for the preparation of medicines. The herbs are combined together in groups of eight, nine, or ten ingredients, packaged in brown paper bags, and dispensed according to written prescriptions by the patients' primary physicians. While there is some contention amongst Chinese physicians on whether herbs or acupuncture should be the primary modality of treatment, Traditional Chinese Medicine—the TCM form of herbology—is being administered almost exclusively to millions of Chinese patients each day. In the form of herbs, TCM is enhancing Qi (the life force) for each Chinese citizen who needs assistance with healing.

In both South America and Central America I studied for weeks at a time with shamans (respected so-called "witch doctors") who were the primary sources of healing for those indigenous people living in the jungles of Belize, Ecuador, Peru, Guatemala, and Panama. When I was in Panama in the spring of 1971, I photographed numerous sources of yellow fever and malaria with only a shaman's herbals as protection against infection. That medicine man's botanicals unquestionably worked well for me. At that time I consulted with tropical disease medical specialists at Panama's Gorgas Hospital, whom I witnessed dispensing some aspects of shaman medicine. In short, much more healing is accomplished worldwide through other methods rather than just from the prescribing of drugs.

Herbal Therapy Is Resurging in the United States

No medicinal claims are allowed for most American herbal products because the U.S. Food & Drug Administration requires the same standard of absolute proof as is required for new synthetic drugs. The FDA has rejected the idea of establishing an independent Expert Advisory Panel for the development of monographs similar to Germany's Commission E monographs, as well as other ideas to create a suitable framework for the marketing of herbal products in the United States. Currently in the United States, herbal products continue to be sold as "food supplements" and manufacturers are prohibited from making any therapeutic claims for their botanical products.[91] Despite this repression, herbal medicine is undergoing a rebirth, as stated, especially in developed countries because scientific researchers are exhibiting a renewed interest. During the last three decades an explosion of herbal information has occurred, which includes crude plant extracts, lesser known pharmaceuticals made from herbs, alkaloids in herbs which heal destabilized DNA, and some highly popular herbal sellers for drug companies which have excited the market.

Finding that it cannot beat down herbal usage by consumers, drug companies have decided to join in with herb product distribution and sale. Currently, over 25 percent of all prescription drugs in the United States contain active constituents obtained from plants. Even codeine and morphine are in this group.

The public, along with their health professionals, are learning that herbs are as useful in treating burns and preventing illness as they are in curing them. The administration of herbal therapy is an example of true holistic medicine in practice, for it deals with the "whole" person by treating the body as an integrated system and not just as a collection of isolated parts.

Beljanski's Anticancer Botanicals as Preventatives

Many dozens of herbal botanicals help the body heal itself and thus act as powerful cancer-prevention treatments. I firmly believe, after having evaluated alternative treatment options for diseases such as cancer in ninety-one published books to date on the subject of natural/non-toxic healing, that the optimal plant therapy in which no evil is done to the body is provided by an individual's ingestion of the botanicals discovered by Mirko Beljanski.

Restoration of a well-functioning DNA is the ultimate in healing, and Beljanski's formulas have proven themselves, both in laboratory studies and in clinical trials, to do exactly that. But because they have also proven themselves to have no side effects on healthy cells, Beljanski's discoveries are invaluable as preventative measures as well, especially if you make the effort to detoxify your body of the external poisons accumulated internally over the years.

To recap the effectiveness of these extracts in terms of prevention, be aware of the following: Each anticancer botanical, Pao pereira and *Rauwolfia vomitoria*, kill cancer cells, and only cancer cells. They don't harm normal healthy cells and have no untoward side effect in the patient.[92] These botanicals may be taken orally, if possible, several times with meals. Since they do not have the same cellular target, ingesting them together gives the patient twice the opportunity to destroy cancer cells. Both can be taken alone as a preventative measure as well as a way to help handle the cancer itself. The synergy these extracts show with conventional treatments means that a combination of the two will have an additive positive effect.

There are certain reasons to select one or the other of these two extracts. *The Rauwolfia vomitoria* has a particular affinity for endocrine tissues (which provide hormones related to breasts, prostate, thyroid, uterus, cervix, ovaries, testes, etc.). Thus the commercial form of this extract is highly desirable for the organs in which hormonal tissues are affected. However, if the patients are receiving hormones, antihormones,

190

or corticoids, *Rauwolfia vomitoria* is not advised since its effect will be neutralized by these medicinal substances.

The *Rauwolfia vomitoria* extract in commercial form is prepared according to Beljanski's procedure, wherein one of its components, alstonine, is concentrated because of its anticancer effects while reserpine is removed to avoid toxicity and side effects. This alkaloid may be ingested by cancer patients in order to fight malignant cells, but it also is a highly effective preventative when a person may be at risk for cancer development. I personally ingest it daily to offset BPH (benign prostatic hyperplasia) which tends to predispose me to prostate cancer. This cancer prevention herbal is additionally useful for women looking to overcome the negative effects of menopause.

Pao pereira fights all cancer cells. It, additionally, has no uncomfortable secondary side effect. This rainforest-grown Pao pereira may be ingested both as a treatment and as a preventative measure. Since this botanical crosses the blood-brain barrier, Pao pereira may increase the beneficial treatments for brain cancer or certain viruses.

Beyond its anticancer activity, Pao pereira strongly inhibits viruses. This antiviral action includes both RNA genome viruses (flu, HIV, FEV, hepatitis C, etc.), and DNA genome viruses (hepatitis A, B, and all of the herpes organisms). Pao pereira, unlike *Rauwolfia vomitoria*, is not modified by hormone usage.

Boosting the Body's Natural Defenses

In chapter 5, I presented to you a brief overview of how Beljanski's RNA primers work. These RNA fragments "prime" (i.e. catalyze or prepare) the duplication of DNA from bone marrow in a very specific manner. Bone marrow cells then physiologically synthesize white blood cells and platelets, restoring the impaired balance for these cells that have been adversely altered by toxic chemicals. RNA fragments make it possible for people undergoing toxic treatments to tolerate them much better and to maintain their bodies' extremely necessary natural immune defenses.[93] This action makes the RNA fragments potentially and naturally preventative in nature.

As the body ages, natural immunity has a tendency to wane, and at least one dose of RNA fragments per week is recommended. Ingesting RNA fragments is also advantageous for people undergoing x-ray examinations or vaccinations which alter the fragile immune cells.

Also in chapter 5, I reported that the special *Ginkgo biloba* extract that Beljanski developed from the golden leaves of that remarkable plant stems from his research in radiation protection. This particular botanical does not resemble other traditional extracts from the same plant, both in terms of its harvest time as well as in its purification and extraction procedures. Beljanski's *Ginkgo* extract was developed to protect people from the dangerous effects of radiation (burns, fibrosis, cicatrix), to improve healing of the skin and tissues in general (wounds, bedsores, scars, etc.), to avoid natural developing fibrosis, and to regulate the function of several proteins and enzymes, impaired either by treatments or by disease.[94]

This *Ginkgo biloba* is particularly recommended for application in certain diseases in which there is an untimely protein build-up—cancer markers, etc.—which make it ideal as a preventative. The excessive protein is both a consequence of cellular deregulation and also a contributing factor in the worsening and continuation of a degenerative disease. Without any known side effects, Dr. Beljanski's extract gives an important boost to the body as it fights to regain internal homeostasis and restore normal health.

Beljanski's botanicals I believe are an important part of any cancer-prevention program for three powerful reasons. They are:

1) selective,

2) immediately eliminative of a small population of cancer cells before tumors develop, which is the paramount goal for any cancer preventative agent, and

3) applicable for periodic ingestion by individuals at high risk or even by healthy elderly or middle-aged people with the aim of stopping prostate cancer, breast cancer, or other cancers before they have a chance to start.

Prevention comes in many forms, and it requires diligence and a willingness to be mindful of what we put into our bodies as well as with what we surround ourselves. Cancer doesn't have to be the dreaded killer that it is reputed to be, but we have to stand up and fight for what we have seen proven scientifically to work against this horrible disease.

Fighting Back Against the Psychology of Fear

Most of us are aware that, for the majority of cancer patients, hearing a diagnosis of "cancer" is the equivalent of receiving a death sentence. Many physicians are well acquainted with the futility of treating patients with the established but often inadequate oncological methods that are usually recommended by our medical institutions. Still these treatments are continually pushed onto medical consumers even when they don't necessarily want them. As I have noted before, conventional cancer treatment is big business. Now the Federal Trade Commission (FTC) is getting active as well.

The FTC is now requiring two random-controlled human trials (RCTs) for any health-related claim that is marketed on a product's label. The cost of such RCTs averages $200,000. In effect, this makes Big Pharma the prime contender because only they can consistently afford the testing required, so only they will be able to produce and sell nutritional supplements with health claims. This new requirement will drive the small manufacturer out of business, and supplements will cost us medical consumers ten times the current price. This announcement was just recently released on May 24, 2011, and Big Pharma is delighted.[95]

The three conventional methods used to treat cancer are: surgery, chemotherapy with toxic drugs, and radiation therapy with X-rays and cobalt radiation. Any other method which might be tried by a holistic-type health-care professional most often is labeled "controversial," "unproven," or "quackery" by the above-mentioned entities.

Even so, a movement is afoot in the United States to change the status quo. Patients are opting out of the conventional system. People who have taken charge of all other aspects of their lives are challenging the powerful bureaucracy which has been able to control the practice of medicine. Instead of seeing themselves as non-powerful patients under the control of those who profess to help but instead harm, these courageous individuals count themselves as "medical consumers." They seek solutions for their health problems in the same way that they manage every other aspect of their lives, by "shopping around." What they discover is that there is a diversity of opinions among medical professionals about how to think about and treat cancer. This "shopping around" is a vital step in fighting back against the psychology of fear which pervades conventional medicine.

The underlying psychology coming from purveyors of conventional cancer treatment is: *do what I tell you to do or you will die.* At that moment, the emphasis shifts from science to business. The patient is no longer facing a scientific decision predicated on the answers to certain questions: *what is cancer and how can I stop what it's doing to my body?* Instead, the patient becomes a customer of the medical (or cancer) industry which makes a profit from the patient's illness. If this industry can control the medical marketplace by gaining a monopoly over the treatment of cancer then their profitability is assured regardless of the merits of their service and/or product. The easiest way for the purveyor of cancer treatments to guarantee their profits is to eliminate any other form of cancer remedy which would compete for their supply of new patients.

Adherents to conventional cancer treatment and the global pharmaceutical companies which profit from the sale of chemotherapy drugs have been able to connive with government officials by means of bribery, awarding of favors, free trips to luxurious places, and all manner of other "gifts." These special favors support the drive for a medical monopoly by legally suppressing medical research and discoveries which would challenge conventional medical therapies. The experience of Dr. Mirko Beljanski in France is just one example of how bureaucratic forces can be manipulated or connived into interfering with scientific progress in favor of Big Pharma business.

As potential cancer patients—for we all are that, no matter how deeply we bury our head in the sand—the real fear in each of our minds should be: *what will happen to me if the forces which continue their drive for a medical monopoly over cancer are victorious?* As politically conscious medical consumers, we must voice our opposition to these monopolistic giants and the bureaucrats which would side with them and prevent the purveyors of conventional cancer treatment from gaining any more control over the medical industry. At the same time, we must work to encourage proper research be done on the most promising alternative methods available so that we can be even better informed about the choices we make.

Dr. Mirko Beljanski devoted his life to discovering the biological tools to fight cancer and infectious viral diseases. Now it is up to us as educated consumers and freedom-loving Americans to fight for what we want and believe is right for us as individuals.

You can do this by seeking out an ACAM physician, a homeopath, or a naturopath and requesting Dr. Beljanski's approach to healing. There are many lifestyle changes which these innovative doctors know to suggest which will improve your health and overall resistance to degenerative and infectious diseases.

The most important first step in fighting back against the terrible psychology of fear that pervades our society in terms of cancer is to take charge of your own health.

The next step is to educate yourself about the tools that are available to you.

The third step is to find a medical professional who understands your personal philosophy and will assist you in accomplishing your goal.

The final step is to speak out, as this book has done, and voice your support for natural and non-toxic botanicals and the right given to you by nature to choose them for yourself.

Case Study: Throat Cancer

From the age of fourteen, Yvon Papineau had earned his living as a professional fisherman in the Bay of Biscay off the southern coast of France between the cities of Bayonne and San Sebastian. Monsieur Papineau (M. Papineau) worked in that capacity for forty-one years until he sold his boat in his fifty-fifth year and took on the role of professional fishing consultant and semi-retired regional supervisor of fisheries. At the time of our interview in September 2003 he was seventy-eight years old and leading the life of a contented, fully retired French gentleman.

Yet, M. Papineau did not always have a life of contentment. Almost eight years before our meeting, it had been predicted by medical specialists that the retired fisherman would be dead within three to six months first because of testicular cancer then because of throat cancer that had been resistant to conventional treatment. Yet, while non-responsive to usual anticancer treatment, the case history of M. Papineau's malignancy is straightforward. He told me about his experience:

"At age seventy, I was keeping myself fit, which was my habit from those past times when I used my strength to haul anchors, lift loaded fish crates, shovel ice, and pull the fish-filled nets on board my boat," says the former fisherman. "During that time following my formal retirement from any kind of work between ages fifty-five to sixty-five, I habitually pedaled a bicycle over country roads for twenty to thirty miles a day. This was just one of the exercises that I practiced regularly. Many other forms of fitness were part of my usual routine.

"One day, after cycling for a full morning, I returned home for lunch and sensed that a pain was affecting my throat when I swal-lowed. So I asked my wife, 'Please look in my mouth; maybe I swallowed a fly or some other insect because it feels like there suddenly is a lump down my throat.' My wife checked inside and saw at the back a white oval object about the size of a pigeon egg," Monsieur Papineau explains. "Before that moment, I had no idea it was lodged there because I never before had felt anything. So the next day I consulted my family physician about the problem.

"After he examined me, our family doctor prescribed an antibiotic on the presumption that I was suffering from an infection. The antibiotic did nothing to take away my discomfort or shrink the throat lump. Thereafter, the doctor suggested that I visit an ear, nose, and throat specialist who also prescribed an antibiotic—a different one. And that prescription didn't give me any relief either. I still had the lump stuck in my throat and now the pain was increasing so much I could no longer ignore it. Upon my return to the throat specialist, he heard my complaint, looked inside my mouth again, observed elsewhere around my head and neck, and plainly stated, 'I'm going to have to operate on your throat because you have a growth down there.'"

M. Papineau's doctor performed surgery and discovered that his patient suffered from a very serious malignancy of the oropharynx, that upper part of the throat that can be seen when one says *Ahhh*. The fisherman's cancer was at Stage III. That meant he had a 10 to 20 percent chance of living five years. The malignancy had metastasized all through his mouth, throat, tonsils, paranasal sinuses, salivary glands, nasopharynx, hypopharynx, larynx, and into other parts of the neck. The medical records indicate that it was improbable this patient would survive beyond twenty weeks.

Although Yvon Papineau never mentioned during the course of our interview that he had been a smoker, it's well-established that almost all cases of oropharyngeal cancer are related to cigarette smoking or pipe smoking or tobacco chewing. Heavy alcohol consumption along with tobacco use further increase the risk.

For oncologists, the preferred conventional treatment involves preoperative chemotherapy, and then surgery combined with post-operative radiotherapy.

"I don't care what the medical books say, I have never smoked in my entire life," M. Papineau told me emphatically. "Nobody in the hospital could determine why or from where my throat cancer arose. The clinicians nevertheless went ahead and gave me post-operative treatment with radiotherapy.

"I underwent twenty radiation treatments for twenty days at three throat [laryngeal] sites," continues M. Papineau. "After that, I underwent six chemotherapy sessions. I was allowed to rest, untreated, for another month when the throat specialist and his colleagues examined me again. It was then that I learned that their treatments were not working, and my prognosis was exceedingly poor. They informed me that I would be dead in three months or at the most would live just six months more.

"What the clinicians did not know is that I had just started taking Dr. Beljanski's products simultaneously while nearing the end of receiving both the radiotherapy and chemotherapy," says M. Papineau. "I did this because my studying of the textbooks on cancer informed me that its conventional ways of treatment with those damned x-ray burnings and chemical poisonings not only would be making me feel awfully sick but also I would be coughing up blood, unable to speak, experiencing burns of the surrounding tissues, losing saliva, having a continuous feeling of dry mouth, lacking appetite, and worse. My reading informed me that Beljanski's supplements—in particular his *Ginkgo* extract—would protect me from all of those negative side effects, and they did. Thus, acting on Beljanski's recommendations, and although the cancer clinicians' burnings and poisonings of my throat tumors did nothing to shrink them, I experienced no negative responses whatsoever.

"My results from using Beljanski's products have been spectacular. I originally took them to counteract any possible side effects from the conventional cancer therapies, but I have continued to swallow Beljanski's supplements because they are keeping me alive and well," Yvon Papineau says. "I have been examined by the very best medical authorities in the Bordeaux area, and these doctors are at a loss to find any reason why I remain in the great shape that they see.

"My throat cancer disappeared at the end of one year after I started on Beljanski's recommended herbs when that tumor should have killed me eight years ago.

"You know what I do to keep myself well? I'll advise you, the same as I've told the doctors: I continue to take Beljanski's supplements and they are responsible for my full recovery with the good health I am experiencing today. Those doctors don't have to scratch their heads in puzzlement wondering why I am still alive. Every day I swallow four capsules of two of Beljanski's anticancer botanicals. The results are there to be seen, and I am still here to be seen." M. Papineau assured me, "Those Beljanski pills are part of my regular daily food supply, and they will remain so as long as I live."

8

Beljanski Remedy Dosages Recorded by French Physician, Christian Marcowith, M.D.

Throughout the prior chapters I have provided pieces of the back story involving the professional jealousy and extreme discord between Mirko Beljanski, Ph.D., and Jacques Monod, Ph.D., Director of the Pasteur institute during most of Beljanski's tenure there. The full narrative of their hatred is the stuff of movies, a story involving interpersonal politics which definitely prevented Dr. Beljanski and his exceedingly important discoveries from receiving their due recognition. The public could have had access much sooner to Beljanski's discoveries concerning cancer and AIDS were it not for the enormous amount of ill will between Beljanski and Monod.

Mirko Beljanski was prohibited from attaining his esteemed rightful place among the world's recognized medical heroes such as Louis Pasteur, Joseph Lister, and Linus Pauling in large part because of the malice felt between Monod and himself. But the stormy tale doesn't stop there. Our intrepid warrior also underwent extreme conflict with the entire French biochemical/pharmaceutical establishment. Contempt and controversy were vigorously pursued against Dr. Beljanski from anyone who utilized drugs and other laboratory-produced, unnatural and toxic-type medical practices against degenerative diseases. Pharmacists, makers of synthetic medicines, and drug distributors were his arch enemies. Those very real conflicts and associated controversies extended from the initial time of Dr. Jacques Monod's administration at the Pasteur

Institute beginning approximately in 1953 to the end of Beljanski's life in 1998 and beyond.

Although the true perception of his genius by the world's scientific community did not actually occur in his lifetime, he is currently acknowledged as a hero. Recognition did arise from medical doctors as well as from his fellow chemical and biological scientists from all around the world. There were numbers of such acknowledgments. One of the most significant tributes paid to the body of work of Dr. Mirko Beljanski is the affirmation offered by practicing French holistic physician Christian Marcowith, M.D. Dr. Marcowith was one of the many very brave medical doctors who prescribed his patients Beljanski's products, even when it was dangerous to do so after the French government had prosecuted Beljanski and found him guilty of practicing medicine illegally.[96]

The Marcowith notes written in French and embodying a variety of health-care practices involving a number of therapies of Complementary, Alternative, Integrative Medicine (CAIM) have already been issued in printed form by EVI Liberty Corporation of New York City with the kind authorization of Dr. Marcowith's widow. They are now available in the published booklet *Cancer: l'Approche Beljanski* (which translates to *Cancer: The Beljanski Approach*).[97]

As Monique Beljanski recalls: "Christian Marcowith was a charming, open, attentive, and discreet man. A native of Isère, France, the region where Mirko had located his privately maintained research laboratory after departing from the Pasteur Institute, Dr. Marcowith was quite familiar with Dr. Beljanski's products. He used them [dispensed to patients from his clinic dispensary] for a long time. The notes [about his treatment results] that Dr. Marcowith left to Mirko are irreplaceable."

This small booklet, *The Beljanski Approach*, produced from the written clinical experiences of Dr. Marcowith, is available only in the French language, and sells in France. I believe an English-language reader who is intent on healing or preventing a degenerative disease can benefit from those reputable holistic medical doctor's treatment notes; they give the required dosage for each of Beljanski's botanicals and his RNA fragments as Dr. Marcowith prescribed for patients to overcome pathologies. Therefore, I am furnishing below a translated version directly from Dr. Christian Marcowith's notebooks and with the blessing of EVI Liberty Corporation.

Dr. Marcowith found, as many others have, that Beljanski's discoveries are *selective*, whether by destroying cancer cells without harming healthy cells or by stimulating the physiological production of beneficial immune cells, or by regulating and normalizing proteins which are built up excessively due to various diseases. Too much protein buildup becomes an accumulated destructive waste that overburdens the body, and that's what Beljanski's botanicals help handle.

Thus below I am providing you with the following translation from the French language of notations made in his own hand by family physician Christian Marcowith, M.D. Dr. Marcowith had a special interest in eliminating degenerative diseases, especially cancers.

> NOTE: This is not advice from a doctor to a patient, nor is it intended to be used as advice from a doctor. These are notes written from one physician to another. As always, seek help from a medical professional when embarking on any treatment for cancer, AIDS, or any other ailment.

Notes from Christian Marcowith, M.D., for Study Purposes on the Discoveries of Mirko Beljanski, Ph.D.

In notebooks assigned for the use of Dr. Mirko Beljanski, Christian Marcowith, M.D., furnished amounts of dosages of all Dr. Beljanski's discoveries, as well as treatment details that he found effective. The information is invaluable for physicians prescribing for patients suffering from any form of cancer or other degenerative diseases such as hepatitis, herpes, HIV, atherosclerosis, prostatitis, and many more.

Dr. Marcowith's notes on therapy for degenerative diseases read as follows:

There are two main anticancer botanicals derived from rain forest herbs, Pao pereira and Rauwolfia vomitoria. *Both kill cancer cells and only cancer cells. They have no toxic effect on the individual. They are taken orally; if possible they should be swallowed several times during the day with meals. As they do not have the same target in the cell, taking them together doubles the individual's chance of destroying cancer cells.*

Both can be used alone as a preventative measure or as a treatment; however, it is important to understand that these two products work in synergy with conventional treatments, meaning that each one maintains its individual mode of action, but the therapeutic effects are compounded. There are two separate reasons to choose one or the other of the botanicals.

Pao pereira fights cancer cells with no side effects. It can be used either as a treatment or as a preventative measure. In addition, the alkaloid in this herb can cross the blood-brain barrier which makes it possible to add it to any treatment protocol for brain cancers and certain viruses. Still, in the latter cases the dose of Pao pereira must be increased since it is only a small fraction of the product that can cross the meningeal barrier.

Other than its anticancer activity, Pao pereira is a strong inhibitor of viruses: in both viruses with RNA genomes such as influenza, HIV, FEV (feline), hepatitis C, etc. as well as DNA genome viruses such as hepatitis A and B and herpes. Pao pereira's effectiveness is not affected by hormones.

Rauwolfia vomitoria *has an affinity for hormonally dependent tissues, including the breasts, prostate, testicles, thyroid, uterus, ovaries, cervix, etc. Thus, this remedy is very desirable if the organ affected is hormonally dependent. Yet, if patients are receiving* hormones, antihormones or corticoids, Rauwolfia vomitoria *is not advised to be taken since its effect will be neutralized by these substances as they compete with one another.* Rauwolfia vomitoria *can be taken to combat the negative effects of menopause, or as a preventative measure in the case of suspicion or risk of a particular pathology.*

RNA fragments from Escherichia coli bacteria [please see Chapter Five on RNA Fragments for a full explanation of this remedy's action] *do not work as an anticancer agent or as an antiviral agent. Instead, the small fragments of RNA are used for stimulating the new and rapid generation of the immune defenses and platelets (thrombocytes), helping patients to better protect themselves from infection. In a situation where conventional cytotoxic therapies* [chemotherapy, radiation therapy, and very serious, traumatic surgery such as in the Whipple's procedure for pancreatic cancer] *have been received, the RNA fragments protect the patients' physiology from such treatments' harsh effects.*

In older people, natural immunity has a tendency to diminish, so the ingestion of one dose per week of small RNA fragments is advised as a preventative measure. One dose is also advised for those people undergoing diagnostic X-ray examinations, vaccinations, etc., which are able to alter the fragile immune cells.

In many auto-immune diseases, there is immunological disorder; therefore, ingesting a few doses of E. coli's small RNA fragments can be quite beneficial. These RNA fragments are taken orally, to be dissolved or melted in the mouth without water.

Beljanski's Ginkgo biloba *is unlike any other conventional plant extract, and so is its application. The unique* Ginkgo biloba *extract is recommended very strongly to anyone undergoing anticancer treatment because disease coupled with conventional treatments work to disrupt normal protein functioning, which poses a danger for the patient. What's more, certain diseases encourage untimely protein buildup, one of the many cancer markers, for example, as well as other cancer markers like gamma GT and transaminases. The* Ginkgo biloba *extract can significantly help to control this process of cancer marker production. In addition, it protects against the fibrosis often induced by radiation over time, as well as the burns that are also associated with radiation treatment.*

Without exhibiting any detrimental side effects, the particular extract of Ginkgo biloba *invented by Beljanski has proven itself to be beneficial to nearly all patients.*

The Protocols as Prescribed for Patients Treated by Christian Marcowith, M.D., using Mirko Beljanski's extracts

The following is the protocol Dr. Marcowith used for patient application of Dr. Beljanski's products against hormonally dependent malignancies. This treatment protocol, recorded in notebooks by Christian Marcowith, M.D., was prescribed by him for patients under his care and was especially useful for those with tumors arising in the endocrine system. The protocol may be applied in conjunction with radiation therapy and/or chemotherapy. In translation from the French, Dr. Marcowith has written:

For Malignancies of the Breast, Prostate, and Uterus

These endocrine system tumors affect organs that secrete specific hormones or growth factors. Here is the protocol for therapeutic application of specific products:

Pao pereira: *swallow 4 to 5 vegetarian capsules per day.*

Rauwolfia vomitoria: *ingest 4 to 5 vegetarian capsules in divided doses, and swallow them three times per day 20 to 30 minutes before each meal. If undertaking any type of hormone treatment using antihormones or corticosteroids, replace the Rauwolfia with Pao pereira (by increasing its dosage).*

Ginkgo biloba: *take 4 to 6 capsules per day*

RNA *fragments from Escherichia coli:* *should be taken if the blood cell levels (white blood cells and platelets) are at reduced levels owing to receiving radiation or chemotherapy. In this case, start taking the RNA fragments the day before any cytotoxic treatments begin.*

The RNA fragments in the form of powders are to be held sublingually [under the tongue] until dissolved, 2 to 3 times per week, and avoid drinking liquids immediately afterwards. Do not ingest RNA fragments close to meal times. Test the patient's blood count often.

The Protocol for Thyroid Cancer

Pao pereira: *ingest 6 to 8 capsules per day*
Rauwolfia vomitoria: *take 4 capsules per day*
Ginkgo biloba: *take 4 capsules per day*
RNA *fragments:* *take the powders according to results of the blood cell count*

The Protocol for Skin Cancer

Pao pereira: *swallow 6 to 8 capsules per day*
Rauwolfia vomitoria: *pop down 4 capsules per day*
Ginkgo biloba: *take 4 to 6 capsules per day*

Application of the Protocol for various Digestive Tract Tumors
Such cancers include:

Carcinoid tumors in the small intestine

In addition to conventional radiation or chemotherapy treatments, take:
Pao pereira: *4 to 8 capsules according to the severity of the situation, plus*

Rauwolfia vomitoria: *4 to 6 capsules per day, plus*
Ginkgo biloba: *4 capsules per day (all the more necessary if undergoing radiation)*

Tumors of the large intestine

With the advent of a strong hormonal response, the risk of intestinal cancer is greatly increased in people with thyroid problems.
In addition to conventional treatment (preferably radiation therapy), take the following:
Pao pereira: *8 to 10 capsules per day during aggressive treatment; 6 to 8 capsules thereafter*
Rauwolfia vomitoria: *4 to 6 capsules per day*
Ginkgo biloba: *4 capsules per day*
RNA fragments *if aplasia* [defective cell count]] *is present: 2 or 3 doses a week*

Esophageal and/or Stomach Cancer

In addition to regular, conventional cytotoxic or radiation treatment, the cancer patient may greatly benefit by taking:
Pao pereira: *6 to 10 capsules per day during aggressive treatment; thereafter reduce to a maintenance dose of 4 to 6 capsules daily*
Rauwolfia vomitoria: *3 to 4 capsules per day*
Ginkgo biloba: *4 to 5 capsules per day*
RNA fragments: *take them if one's reduced level of white blood cells or platelets necessitates such ingestion.*

Pancreatic Cancer

This is an extremely difficult malignancy to overcome inasmuch as it has a mere 1.5 percentage rate of survival for up to five years.
In addition to conventional treatments (generally radiation therapy and/or chemotherapy), take:

Pao pereira: *10 capsules or more each day*
Rauwolfia vomitoria: *5 capsules per day*
Ginkgo biloba: *6 to 8 capsules per day*
Monitor transaminase and GT gamma, which are cancer markers indicating the cancer's evolution.

Brain Tumors

In addition to radiation therapy, the cancer patient may benefit from the fact that the active ingredient in the Pao pereira extract crosses the meningeal barrier and shows a synergy of action with radiation therapy that fights this type of cancer and, more generally, all brain cancers. Pao pereira's equally antiviral action will allow it to fight certain viruses which induce brain cancers.
Pao pereira: *take 8 to 12 capsules per day*
Ginkgo biloba: *swallow 4 to 6 capsules per day. This herb is made all the more necessary in the case of radiation therapy in order to avoid the fibrosis caused by radiation waves.*

Myeloma, Leukemia

A three-pronged approach may be advantageous:

*A – **Pao pereira** extract acts in synergy with conventional treatments to strengthen the inhibition of malignant cells and/or the inhibition of viruses, which we know often play a role in the formation of malignant hemopathies.*
For the aggressive phase: Swallow 2 Pao pereira capsules per 22 lbs. of body weight per day (approximate). Then: reduce the dosage to 1 capsule per 22 lbs. of body weight per day (approximate). Capsules to be taken before breakfast and dinner.
*B – **RNA fragments** preserve normal bone marrow cell replication and, therefore, stimulate immunity: ingest 1 dose every other day during chemotherapy and two doses per week outside of treatments.*

The number of platelets must also be monitored each week and dosage should be increased if necessary (maximum: 3 doses per week).

In a case where correction of aplasia is the required objective (for example in acute leukemia), start taking RNA fragments only after obtaining aplasia in order to accelerate the regeneration of leukocyte populations.

Ferritin, a protein that stores iron, forms as a result of the damage caused to erythrocytes [red blood cells] *by chemotherapy. It enters the bone marrow mostly from the liver and spleen and prevents the formation of red blood cells. One needs 2.7 million red blood cells to ensure sufficient oxygenation for syntheses and to ensure that RNA fragments can work effectively. However, when RNA fragments are given to a patient with low red blood cell counts, it helps him to avoid complications. The medical technician can do a red blood cell transfusion and then give the RNA fragments which will immediately start to work; one will then note the increase in leucocytes* [white blood cells] *and platelets.*

The addition of magnesium makes it possible to curb the excess of ribonucleases in the patient's plasma.

Cytotoxic agents used for chemotherapy invariably are accompanied by unwanted adverse side effects. For instance, response to chemotherapy is very often accompanied by malignant cell resistance and resistance of certain enzymatic dysfunctions. In these cases, one particular Beljanski remedy works well. It is:

C – **Ginkgo biloba** *helps to regulate the activity of numerous enzymes. The administration of this herb is straightforward: Take 2 capsules of Dr. Beljanski's unique* Ginkgo *extract in the morning and evening starting at the beginning of chemotherapy treatment.*

Bone Cancer

Bones afflicted by cancerous tumors lose calcium and phosphate. These two minerals tend to form a combined coating which covers the tumor and protects it against the effects of natural extracts. Yes, after cauterization with radiation, the tumor will once again be treatable.
Pao pereira: *ingest 8 to 10 vegetarian capsules per day.*
Ginkgo biloba: *take 4 per day.*
RNA *fragments* *should be taken during radiation therapy.*

The Lymphoma Cancers

Skin lymphoma

Pao pereira: *swallow 3 capsules of the herbal remedy morning and evening, 20 minutes before mealtime.*
Rauwolfia vomitoria: *swallow 2 to 3 capsules per day of this herbal extract (as much for its cumulative effect as for its florescent marker effect) and also because this anticancer remedy has to do with hormonally dependent tissues (by means of testosterone).*

Non-Hodgkin's lymphoma

Pao Pereira: *take 8 to 10 capsules per day (during aggressive treatment with radiation therapy).*
Ginkgo biloba: *take 4 to 6 capsules per day.*
RNA *fragments*: *ingest according to blood cell levels (to be adjusted).*

Hodgkin's lymphoma

Pao pereira: *ingest 8 to 10 capsules per day of Pao Pereira.*
Ginkgo biloba: *take 4 to 6 capsules per day of this herb.*

Ideal Duration of Treatment with Dr. Beljanski's Products

Pao pereira *and* **Rauwolfia vomitoria:** *take these two inhibitor extracts together for their synergistic effect.*

a. *Start as early as possible following diagnosis.*

b. *Take the supplements over the course of the day, before breakfast and dinner.*

c. *Continue, concurrent with other traditional therapies, until the clinical state has once again become satisfactory. To be prudent, one can continue with the Beljanski extracts for a month or two past this point.*

d. *Later, engage in cyclical usage for preventative purposes from 2 to 5 months per year.*

For the two Beljanski remedy regulators

RNA fragments:
Start just after chemotherapy or radiation treatments have begun when they are inducing a drop in white blood cells (unless aplasia is the objective). Continue until white blood cells and platelets have returned to normal. Take one dose preferably sublingually, one to three times per week. Do not drink any liquid immediately afterward. Ideally the RNA fragments are to be taken under the tongue far from mealtimes.

If the patient is taking heparin: ingest RNA fragments either twelve hours before or twelve hours after use of this drug.

Ginkgo biloba:
In order to regulate/curb hyperactivity of certain enzymes; synergistic usage of this herb is used with traditional cytotoxic treatments. To fight radiation burns: start preferably just before ionizing treatments are received that may induce fibrosis; continue until the end of radiation treatments, even up to a

month afterwards. Previous fibroses may also be advantageously treated. The sooner the strategies are implemented, the better the results.

Cancer Prevention

(Author's note: while I have delved into the subject of cancer prevention in the preceding chapter, I am including Dr. Marcowith's notes on prevention, for they reiterate important information.)

Pao pereira *and* **Rauwolfia vomitoria** *extracts have no side effects and do not cause resistance to developing healing effects. In the absence of cancerous cells to attach themselves to, the molecules of alkaloid present within the two herbs (the actual healing agents) are rapidly eliminated from the body since they only join themselves to deregulated cells. Consequently, these extracts can easily be taken as a means of prevention in all precancerous states. One can also use them in recurrent cycles as a means of prevention in people with high risk of developing cancer.*

RNA fragments, *in the same way, can be ingested with no toxicity as a means of prevention/repair for chromosomal breakage that inevitably accompanies ionizing radiation examinations (mammography, scintigraphy, X-rays, etc.). Take one cone-shaped unit of RNA fragments 24 hours before the examination and another one day after.*

Further Advice

Exposure to the sun is never recommended because UV rays stimulate the multiplication of cancerous and viral cells. A diet excessively rich in iron (which includes red meat, lentils, parsley) is not recommended for anyone afflicted with cancer or a viral illness. Iron stimulates multiplication of cancerous and viral cells. It can also disturb the activity of certain enzymes.

(For the ideal diet to prevent ingesting Ferritin from an excessive intake of iron, please see *The Gerson Therapy: The Amazing Nutritional Program for Cancer and Other Illnesses* about cancer treatment strictly using diet and nutritional supplementation.[98] Please also view the information for Charlotte Gerson and The Gerson Institute description and location in Appendix A.)

An excess of molecular calcium (Ca++) can be dangerous to certain sensitive lymphocyte lines, and intake of this mineral should be controlled if the lymphocyte level is too low. Again, please see a qualified doctor for more information and advice about this issue.

Taking magnesium in reasonable doses is always advisable for those afflicted with AIDS or cancer. Not only the illness but also the chemotherapy and radiation therapy treatments modify and strengthen the nuclease activity in the blood. Magnesium and Ginkgo biloba *make it possible to reduce this excessive activity. Selenium and riboflavin are not to be missed either. Monitor these two nutrients, inasmuch as too small an amount of selenium facilitates cirrhosis of the liver.*

Zinc should also be monitored in cases of cancer or AIDS. The blood level of this mineral should remain normal. Too little or too much zinc leads to disturbances in the lymphocyte levels. If there is excessive zinc, lower it through the interplay of copper and magnesium in measured doses. Avoid foods rich in zinc (i.e. oysters, wheat germ, yeast, dairy products). Do not lose sight of the fact that a zinc diet leads to a decrease in catalase activity (one of the major enzymes used in food digestion) in the kidneys and liver. If there is not enough zinc, take extra zinc supplementation (zinc orotate is quite easily assimilated). Swallow zinc supplements in measured doses two times per day. Keep close watch as this mineral increases and stop when it has reached normal levels.

An excess of copper can lead to zinc deficiency. To neutralize copper, prescribe zinc in measured doses for about one month.

If someone must take hormones, antihormones or corticoids for a lengthy period of time, abstain from taking Rauwolfia vomitoria *because these molecules will reduce its effects. In this case, replace* Rauwolfia vomitoria *with Pao pereira.*

It is preferable to exclude any gastro-intestinal dressings that contain clay or aluminum. (In other words, whenever you're dealing with gastro-intestinal issues, do not use clay or aluminum.)

In all circumstances where the level of ferritin is shown to be high, avoid ingesting extra vitamin C. Ferritin blocks the formation of hemoglobin in the liver and bone marrow and weakens red blood cells. As the degradation of red blood cells releases iron, ferritin increases. Especially monitor the patient undergoing several blood transfusions. When there are repeated transfusions, think about the antibodies able to destroy blood cells (white blood cells and platelets). The antibodies destroy the blood cells as soon as the RNA fragments can generate them.

Insulin does not interfere with these products developed by Dr. Beljanski.

Heparin administered intravenously can prevent RNA fragments from working. Take RNA fragments and heparin at different times, separated by twelve hours, before or after.

Repeated mammographies and echographies can lead to chromosomal destabilization. Their repair is facilitated by taking RNA fragments one or two hours before the exam.

During radio-isotopic exploration (scintiscanning, mammography, measure of organ output with radioactive markers, synoviorthese, etc.), give RNA fragments a couple of hours before each test in order to protect against chromosomal breakage.

For rare patient situations in which RNA fragments are not sufficiently effective, include the following additional bits of advantageous information: either a lack of hemoglobin (fewer than 2.5 million red blood cells), or an excess of ribonuclease (this last case is able to be mitigated in part by taking magnesium).

An especially significant point for slightly anemic people is that Dr. Marcowith records the following in his notes: *Having fewer than 2.5 million red blood cells causes a release of ferritin and a considerably slowed synthesis of white blood cells and platelets. Ferritin enters the bone marrow and the liver, preventing the synthesis of hemoglobin, a situation which considerably blocks the efficacy of RNA fragments. It is therefore necessary to start treatment by raising the level of red blood cells.*

Extensive Recognition for Mirko Beljanski, Ph.D., Received from His Scientific Peers

During his lifetime Mirko Beljanski, fluent in his native Serbian, in French, and in English, was invited to present his work throughout the world. Dr. Beljanski's papers were published in many peer-reviewed national, international and highly-respected scientific journals (please see Appendix A for the full list of Mirko Beljanski's 133 scientific publications). Dr. Jacques Monod's opposition to Dr. Beljanski publishing in French turned out to be somewhat fortunate for it became an opportunity for greater international exposure and worldwide recognition.

In the book that she dedicated to her husband, Monique Beljanski published letters spanning several decades which reflected his peer's respect and esteem for the research he conducted.[99] Monique provided me with some of these letters for publication here. For instance, as early as 1973, Armin C. Braun of Rockefeller University in New York City wrote (in part) in a letter:

Dear. Dr. Beljanski:
I read with great interest your manuscript on transforming RNA in crown gall [a plant disease]. I find this work very exciting and I would urge you to publish it at the earliest possible time in a journal that has a wide circulation such as the Proceedings of the National Academy of Sciences, Nature, or Science. You appear to have made a very important discovery and have obtained for the first time the sterile induction of transportable crown gall tumors with a specific agent other than bacteria.

In the 1980s following Beljanski's visit to Howard University in Washington D.C., Associate Director of Research Kenneth Olden, Ph.D., and Seminar Committee Chairman Sandra L. White, Ph.D., wrote to Dr. Beljanski saying: "We, as well as our associates, were greatly inspired by your presentation. With the continued support of committed individuals like yourself, we are convinced that we can build a 'first-rate' research operation here at Howard."

Echoing this excitement over Beljanski's research, Swedish researcher Sten Friberg, M.D., Ph.D., contacted Dr. Beljanski following the presentation of one of his papers, exclaiming: "Your ideas and results are simply fascinating."

In the 1970s and 1980s before Dr. Jacques Monod's wrath succeeded in isolating Dr. Mirko Beljanski and turned him into a scientific black sheep, several renown big wigs in the French medical community, such as Professor Bernard Halpern, M.D., (of the Institute of Immune Biology, Paris, France), dared to praise Beljanski, saying [translated]: "Your work is of extreme importance for which I congratulate you. It deserves an award from the Academy of Sciences."

In 1988, the Oncology Clinic at the Bobigny University Hospital was conducting an experiment on Dr. Beljanski's *Ginkgo biloba* extract (named Bioparyl at the time) and its effectiveness in treating fibrosis. After obtaining positive results, the clinic's researchers sent Dr. Beljanski the following letter, in which they stated [translated]:

"As per your request, here are the preliminary results we have obtained in the post-radiation lesions following treatment with Bioparyl. It is still too early to ascertain the effect of dosage. However, its effectiveness is evident, especially in the current stage of our experiment, in cutaneous and mucus membrane fibroses."

For anyone familiar with human nature, it is not at all surprising that domestic support for Beljanski ended as the French government increased its efforts to silence and censure him. In the face of this mounting pressure, the continuous support and demonstration of friendship from Research Scientist Maurice Stroun from Geneva University in Switzerland is even more remarkable. Professor Stroun, as you will see in the following letter, did not hesitate to express his indignation to the French prosecutor who had issued the warrant for Beljanski's arrest. In this letter, Dr. Stroun remarkably summarized what "crimes" his friend, Dr. Mirko Beljanski, committed and explains the wrath of the French establishment. Dr. Stroun interviewed with me in Paris and verbalized what he wrote in his letter. I believe that it is appropriate here to reproduce this extraordinary letter in part, but I wish I could have the entire document, for it holds the full and flourishing signature of Professor in Biochemistry Maurice Stroun, Ph.D., from the University of Geneva, in Switzerland. The letter:

Professor Maurice Stroun, Ph.D.
University of Geneva

> The Honorable Judge Anne TARELLI
> High Court of Créteil
> Pasteur Vallery-Radot Street
> 91011 Créteil
>
> Geneva, October 21st, 1996

Dear Madam:

I would like to express how appalled I am at how Professor Mirko Beljanski has been, and is being, treated.

What crime has he committed?

> a) The crime of being a great researcher, who shed light on a very special characteristic of tumor cell DNA structure, among other things? Thanks to this characteristic, he demonstrated that with a certain alkaloid (whose name and whose preparation are

described in the patent he took out and which is thus available to the public), [Dr. Morton Walker's note: this alkaloid's name is Flavopereirine] animal tumors can be blocked to a very significant degree. In a Geneva University Hospital laboratory, it was shown that this alkaloid blocked human cancer cell lines that had been resistant to other chemotherapy products.

b) The crime of making it possible for us to make an important discovery in the field of cancer screening? In effect, Dr. P. Anker and I just made a discovery laying the foundation for a non-invasive method for detecting cancer in the blood plasma of cancer patients. At the beginning of our research, we used Beljanski's discovery concerning the specific nature of the structure of cancer cell DNA. As you may know, in September of this year our work was praised by the most prestigious medical reviews as an important advancement in the field of oncology.

I understand that certain scientific, and especially political, personalities connected to the Health Ministry are troubled. What would become of their work if work in the U.S.A. confirms the importance of Beljanski's discoveries? It would be better to give him his walking papers, meaning arrest him, forbid him from continuing his research, and confiscate his passport so that he can no longer contact his American colleagues. It would be better to give walking papers to all those doctors who were so snide as to think that it is more important for their patients to live by breaking the established medical rules than to die by submitting to them…

…I admit that I have advised cancer and HIV positive patients to consult doctors willing to give prescriptions allowing them to use PB-100 [Pao pereira], without foregoing other treatments, except in terms of AZT. Besides, perhaps the one explains the other. If I, or a member of my family, had one of these two diseases, as a biologist fully informed as to PB-100's action, I would take it or have them take it.

Signed by Dr. Maurice Stroun

I think Professor Stroun speaks for all of us who have studied and used Dr. Beljanski's products. My hope is that they will one day become widely accepted as effective treatments by themselves and in conjunction with conventional treatments so that no one need suffer from the ill-effects of cancer treatments anymore.

9

A Lasting Legacy

Our extraordinary hero, Dr. Mirko Beljanski, died a most heartbreaking death in his home on October 28th, 1998. He succumbed to acute myeloid leukemia, a cancer that he may have treated with his own botanicals, had he had access to them.

Power takes on many forms, and it could be argued that Dr. Beljanski was simply a hard-working and honest pawn in a much larger chess game of power and money played out by the dealings of the large pharmaceutical industry in league with a too-complicit French government. As Dr. Stephen Coles points out in his book on Beljanski's life, *Extraordinary Healing*, the French government and pharmaceutical industry have a long history of "working hand-in-hand against natural and non-toxic therapies."[100] That coupled with the long-standing animosity against Beljanski exhibited by Dr. Jacques Monod and his successors at the Pasteur Institute, J.P. Aubert, the director for the Department of Biochemistry and Microbial Genetics, and F. Gros, general director, both of whom shared Monod's likes and dislikes especially in people, made the climate in which Beljanski worked tense at best. Indeed, as I reported in chapter 6, Beljanski's findings on HIV and other viruses were kept out of the public eye because of the potential controversy surrounding the findings.

Since when do politics and power grabs get in the way of science finding ways to make life better for humankind? It unfortunately happens all the time, and Beljanski's life can only be compared to a Greek tragedy: a towering genius, working against all odds to find a cure for two of the most dreaded diseases in modern history, struck down and eventually eliminated by the very forces charged with protecting the public interests. But just as the lessons of the great Greek dramas have survived throughout the ages, the work of this great scientist and humanitarian has survived practically against all odds.

Beljanski's Lab Raided

In France, identical to the way drug consumers are exploited in the United States, a powerful and well-financed pharmaceutical industry claiming to protect the public's welfare possesses the political and financial means to oppress health professionals who prescribe botanicals which embody the CAIM (Complementary, Alternative, and Innovative Medicine) philosophy. As far back as 1989, members of the French government were working to find ways to stop Beljanski from carrying on his research and helping those afflicted with cancer and AIDS with his botanicals. Dr. Coles reports that one Claude Evin, the minister of social affairs and health at the time, "filed charges of illicit practice of medicine against Beljanski."[101] The court that had jurisdiction over Beljanski's private laboratory at the time decided that the good doctor was not guilty of practicing medicine illegally, but that didn't stop those who wanted to take Beljanski down. Beljanski's discoveries were actually keeping people alive. Such results represented a direct threat to the bottom line of the government's beloved pharmaceutical industry.

As I noted in chapter 4, in late 1993 and into 1994, the French government ordered additional tests of what it deemed to be the Pao pereira extract, labeled at the time as PB-100. The results came up negative. The product that was tested did not exhibit anti-viral properties, but many, including Beljanski's wife, believe that somehow either the substance was altered or the test was set up to fail. In fact, another test set up by the former head of the Institute for Medicine at the University of Bern in Switzerland, theoretically using the same materials as tested in the French trial, showed that PB-100 did, indeed, have anti-viral properties. [102]

Perhaps all this animosity and foul play was exacerbated by the fact that the Beljanski team had applied and was most likely very close to receiving approval from the *Autorisation de Mise sur le Marche* (the AMM), the French equivalent of the U.S. Food and Drug Administration. Doctors across western Europe continued to prescribe the formulas, but the authorities were closing in on Beljanski, seeking to shut him down because he was cutting into their profits and tarnishing their credibility. Then a small miracle happened. The then President of France, François Mitterrand, suffering from acute prostate cancer, was all but given up for dead by his political opponents and the French press when he started taking Beljanski's botanicals. I have already reported on this story in the introduction, but I repeat it here because as long as Mitterrand was alive, the government couldn't touch the beleaguered researcher and his team.[103]

Finally, after a relapse of almost two years, the French president's cancer got the best of him, and he died January 8, 1996. The *Autorisation de Mise sur le Marche* was close to putting their stamp of approval on the Beljanski formulas but his enemies were too swift. On October 9, 1996, at 6 a.m., the *Groupe d'Intervention de la Gendarmerie Nationale* (the National Gendarmerie Intervention Group), or GIGN, raided Beljanski's laboratory. The GIGN is the arm of the French special forces whose missions include the arrest of armed criminals, in particular those taking hostages, counter-terrorism, and dealing with aircraft hijacking, and ending prison riots. Sending in the GIGN was clearly overkill, and it indicated the order came from the highest level of government.[104]

During my September 2003 visit to La Rochelle, France, I spoke with a number of former staff members of the Beljanski research team who were at the lab when it was raided. They reported that soldiers and police appeared to be conducting a war and behaved as if in combat. I learned that the military squadron, basically a SWAT team, acted as if these ordinary French citizens, possessing no weapons and with no criminal history, were the worst kind of terrorists. These so-called "terrorists" of course were simply Beljanski's laboratory staff members—about a dozen—who were frightened into complete paralysis.

With their helicopter overhead surveying the place, whistles blowing, German Shepherd guard dogs lunging at the end of leashes, warnings broadcasted over bull horns, this SWAT-like team, wearing flack vests and waving drawn guns, conducted their invasion on Beljanski's research facilities with malicious vigor. In this manner, for more than an hour, the squad of military police disassembled Dr. Beljanski's entire laboratory building. They forced open locked closets, broke into cupboards, confiscated computers and notebooks, removed nutrients and medicines, and herded together rabbits, guinea pigs, and mice.

Can you imagine the horror of confronting federal agents appearing unannounced on your doorstep, armed with machine guns, demanding access to laboratory glassware, microorganism records, experimental animals, medical equipment, and work-bench supplies as mundane as rubber gloves, treating the entire laboratory facility as a crime scene? Might you be shocked by seeing your diplomas, award certificates, and hanging pictures seized from the walls? Would you find it even worse witnessing more agents showing up at your private residence, again carrying machine guns, pistols, and rifles, demanding that your spouse open the door for a full search of your sleeping quarters? Could you conceive of the police helping themselves to your computers both in your work place and at home? Is it possible for you to mentally grasp what's happening when you watch them carting away whatever they choose, with no copies left?

To this day, the French Government has not yet returned most of the confiscated property which encompasses Dr. Beljanski's entire life's work, including his laboratory equipment, hand-written notebooks and typed records, computers and office furniture, Petri dishes filled with growing specimens, and stocks of therapeutic substances such as herbs from overseas. Perhaps most important of all, the French Government still holds in its possession the file for *Demande d'autorisation sur le*

Marché (the marketing authorization application for the supplements that was close to being approved). The French military personnel chained the doors shut and permanently closed Dr. Beljanski's personal research facility, and all without any due process of law. His staff was not permitted even to retrieve their personal items.

Shortly after, Dr. Mirko Beljanski, seventy-three years old, was humiliatingly roused from bed, arrested, and taken to the local prison where he was held for twenty-four hours without questioning and a bail that was set so high he couldn't possibly have paid it.[105] Worse, he was not given any information about what he was being charged with nor was he advised of his rights. I have no doubt that if the Bastille were still standing, he would have been unceremoniously thrown into the deepest part of the dungeon with the worst of the other political prisoners and left there to rot. (The Bastille was the infamous French prison that housed not only common criminals but people deemed dangerous to the state. The storming of the Bastille, in which commoners demanded the release of all prisoners, marks the beginning of the French Revolution.)

Monique, his wife, was put under house arrest in their small apartment in Paris and was not allowed to use the phone to ask for legal advice, nor was she given any information about her husband. Worse, before the standard due process of the law could take over, which would have allowed for charges to be made, evidence to be presented, and a chance for Beljanski to defend himself, the French Assistant Attorney General's Office ordered the destruction of all Beljanski's products. The police then went to the AMM and confiscated all of the documents concerning the filing for market authorization.

Under threat of further imprisonment, Dr. Beljanski was forced to discontinue his forty-five years of work in life science and instruct his laboratory employees to go home and keep their mouths shut so that they would not have additional penalties heaped upon them. Worse, the court ordered that all Beljanski products be removed from the homes of those who were taking them. The French authorities, according to

Dr. Coles, using information gained from doctors, made their way from home to home, terrorizing ordinary French citizens, and confiscating their botanicals. It was an egregious violation of basic civil and criminal rights, and it was made worse by the fact that Dr. Beljanski was unable to defend himself, for he had been deprived of the basic right to plead his case before an impartial judge. It was injustice heaped on injustice. Another decree was issued stating that he was not allowed to speak publicly, was not allowed to publish his research, and in the most flagrant violation of the right to free speech, was not allowed to write for the press. Patients, outraged that their botanicals had been taken from them, took to the streets in Paris and Lyons to fight for their right to use the supplements that were saving their lives.[106]

This true tale of political intrigue and corruption in France is likely the reason why information about Beljanski's discoveries has not been more widespread. Furthermore, I've concluded that ultimately, the French Government is likely to have contributed to Dr. Beljanski's premature death. Informed persons know that such an overtaxing burden of the magnitude experienced by Dr. Mirko Beljanski can be deadly.

In a cruel irony, in part due to stress from the inglorious actions of his nation's government, Dr. Beljanski contracted the same illness he so successfully fought against in others. Although at seventy-four, his chances were very limited, but he might have saved himself from the agony of dying from the acute form of leukemia that took over his body if he would have had access to his own supplements, products he spent a lifetime developing.

As befits the plot of a Greek tragedy, instead of the acclaim he deserved, the elder Dr. Beljanski was hounded by jealous associates, competitive drug executives, and zealous bureaucrats who prevented him from presenting his marvelous discoveries to the world and saving lives sooner rather than later.

The Last Discovery

But while the French government was able to kill the man, they will never be able to take away the body of research he left behind. Mirko Beljanski, who during the course of his life was driven by a passion for knowledge (be it in biochemistry, pathology or evolution), also made a beautiful discovery near the very end of his career and fortunately was able to publish his findings. The science of it, of course, is complicated, but the gist of it is Dr. Beljanski was close to discovering the very origins of life. He was able, through many years of research, to recreate DNA from scratch. It's called *de novo* synthesis. *De Novo* is a Latin term which means "created a new" and implies "without a template, without a model, a synthesis from simple elements." In other words, he was able to create DNA out of simple elements that he and others believed to have existed on earth billions of years before life appeared.

DNA, that exceptional molecule of life, has a mysterious origin. No one knows exactly how over the course of evolution this molecule—able to repair itself, replicate, and correctly transmit all the characteristics of a living being—came to exist. Its spontaneous formation seems impossible.[107]

Dr. Beljanski, like many other microbiologists, have long been drawn to the question of the origin of life. What has confounded researchers is that spontaneous production of DNA is a classic "chicken and egg" paradox. Proteins are responsible for synthesizing nucleic acids, yet it takes the DNA and RNA to tell the cell which amino acids to put together to form that protein. Which one came first? At some point, long ago in biological evolution, this very complex DNA molecule was formed. But how?

Using the same enzyme (PNPase) that Dr. Ochoa discovered in the 1950s when the Beljanskis worked with him at New York University, Dr. Beljanski was able to create a DNA strand that did exactly what DNA should do—replicate itself and the genetic code it contains.

This was the phenomena he was researching up until the raid on his laboratory, and it is in keeping with the caliber of scientist that he was. Many of the best natural scientists have been known to turn their attention to philosophical issues as they near their careers' termination. The physicist Erwin Schrödinger, Ph.D., for example, famous for the role his imaginary cat played in quantum mechanical theory, published his lectures in a volume called *What Is Life?*[108] His collection has been interpreted as predicting the genetic function of DNA. Christian DeDuve gave an account of the major events throughout evolution in his book popular among scientists and consumers alike, *Blueprint for a Cell: The Nature and Origin of Life.*[109]

Beljanski's last publication reported the results of an experiment he had worked on for many years, but in it, and typical of all of his work, he avoided philosophizing and instead clearly addressed one of the most fundamental problems in the evolution of life. He stated that it took the presence of iron for the enzyme PNPase to synthesize DNA. His new finding, as with many others described in the book you are reading now, have been ignored by the scientific and medical mainstreams.

I couldn't agree more with the eminent Swiss biologist, Dr. Maurice Stroun, who said emphatically to me, "Mirko's discoveries must be re-discovered!" Dr. Stroun's stated notion is what I am attempting to do by getting this book published, read, and its information acted upon. Such constructive movements will not only inspire new generations of researchers but will potentially save multi-millions of lives. Of that I am certain.

A Daughter's Homage

Dr. Mirko Beljanski and his work could have suffered the fate of obscurity if it weren't for the firm tenacity with which his daughter and wife pursued his legacy.

Mirko Beljanski was martyred by the French government. He spent his life bucking what was fashionable, pioneering research that the establishment feared and thus dismissed.

As he recognized that his death was imminent, Beljanski painstakingly went over his life's work with his daughter, Sylvie, who diligently transferred all the information to which he still had access to America, where they hoped medical freedom still existed. His goal was to put his life's work into "easy-to-understand language so that more people would access it." [110] Finally, he requested that he be taken off all treatments so he could return home to die.

Sylvie Beljanski's outstanding commitment to carry on with her father's legacy has led to a number of remarkable events and inspired others to further achievements, which are becoming themselves part of the exceptional story.

Starting with my trip to France to collect the testimonies from cancer and HIV survivors and write this book, I was moved by the dedication of all those men and women who traveled to the CIRIS picnic to share with complete strangers how they were able to overcome sickness and offer their own recovery as a beacon of hope to others. Other journalists and photographers have also felt compelled to report these remarkable stories, and I am told that a fifty-minute documentary movie has been filmed.

Since Dr. Beljanski's death, lawyers have felt energized to fight for justice and try to undo, one by one, the wrong done against Mirko and Monique Beljanski. As a result, these two who were totally unprepared for litigation because of their mindset exclusively on science, were in the end again and again vindicated by the courts. In 1994, when Beljanski was accused of practicing medicine without a license, in an unprecedented move, the General Attorney put aside his papers and pleaded himself for a non-guilty verdict. After years of *pro bono* work, a French tax attorney got a Court of Appeal to side with Monique Beljanski and the French IRS dropped their unjustified request of more than 1 million Euros (about 1.5 million dollars).

After his death, his daughter, a lawyer, with the help of her mother, brought a case against France to the European court of Human Rights. On May 23, 2002, the court issued a decree claiming that Mirko Beljanski had been "denied a fair trial and the opportunity to defend his legacy and the scientific value of his research." Moreover, the high court found *unanimously* that Beljanski's "right to be granted a fair trial in a reasonable time frame had been seriously violated."[111] Beljanski's surviving family won a small cash damage claim in the lawsuit against their country in the name of Mirko Beljanski, and they used the cash settlement to set up a foundation in their father's name, the Beljanski Foundation.

I am happy to report that CIRIS along with the Beljanski Foundation's work on both sides of the Atlantic are engendering global interest in Mirko Beljanski. Exciting research projects involving other institutions are currently in the works. But in the end, the goal for Sylvie today is the same as it was for Mirko forty years ago. Although she is not working in the laboratory, she is still continuing his mission to educate people about the danger that environmental toxins present to health and to encourage them to look for ways to take charge of their own health.

Her message stresses the importance of detoxification, the elimination of heavy metals and toxins that make the bed for debilitating conditions and over time gradually destabilize the secondary structure of the DNA's double helix. The Beljanski legacy has now spanned continents and generations. But Sylvie, who speaks constantly at conferences globally about her father's research and environmental toxins, says emphatically to anyone who will listen, "There is still so much left to do!"

I can hear echoes of her father in that last battle cry, and I cannot think of a better legacy for a daughter to leave her father.

A Final Tribute

One of the purposes of this book is to rescue Dr. Beljanski's life's work from obscurity and present it to a world-wide audience of needy victims of illness. Additionally it is my heart-felt intention that somehow Mirko Beljanski will finally be awarded the professional recognition that he assuredly deserves. This book is also a call for the French Government to publically redress the gross injustice that Dr. Beljanski suffered due to its vindictive bureaucrats' destructive excesses. The government of France has served its people and the rest of our world poorly, and it deserves censorship.

Dr. Mirko Beljanski could have lived a life of obscurity, a poor farmer tending his geese and pigs. He certainly was in danger of being long forgotten after his death, his research and his botanicals buried away in a filing cabinet in some musty old government building in Paris. But I have found in my long years as a medical researcher that great and lasting discoveries may remain hidden for a while, but they will all eventually see the light of day. The human spirit is indomitable. We do not want to condemn ourselves to lives of needless suffering, and the truth, as they say, will win out in the end.

There *is* hope for those who suffer from all those deadly diseases whose cures remain elusive. The German philosopher, Arthur Schopenhauer, once said, "All truth passes through three stages. First, it is ridiculed. Second, it is violently opposed. Third, it is accepted as being self-evident."

Dr. Mirko Beljanski's ideas were once ridiculed by his peers. They were certainly violently opposed by the French government and their close cohorts, Big Pharma. With more research to validate the forward-looking microbiologist's work, I know with certainty that in my lifetime, I will see Dr. Mirko Beljanski's botanicals accepted as a self-evident cure for cancer.

Notes to Preface

[1] *The Merck Manual of Medical Information*, Second Home Edition, "Cancer of the Pancreas." Mark H. Beers, M.D., Editor-in-Chief, Merck Research Laboratories, Whitehouse Station, NJ, Diagnosis Section, 2003, P. 774.

[2] Morgan, G., R. Ward, and M. Barton. "The contribution of cytotoxic chemotherapy to 5-year survival in adult malignancies." *Clinical Oncology* 2004, 16 (80:549-560).

[3] *Dr. Julian Whitaker's Health & Healing*® published by Healthy Directions, LLC., Vol. 21, No. 3, March 2011, P. 1.

Notes to Introduction

[4] CIRIS is an acronym that stands for the *Centre d'Innovations, de Recherches et d'Informations Scientifiques*, (Center of Scientific Innovations, Research, and Information). Led by Mme. Pierrette Weidlich and whose activities are located mainly in Europe, CIRIS works with the Beljanski Foundation and sponsors research and clinical trials testing Beljanski® products.

In the context of the national and international laws that govern the Public Health Association, who acts as an international civic Non-Governmental Organization (O.N.G.), CIRIS has several aims which are listed on the website. Please see www.Beljanski.com.

CIRIS also periodically publishes a limited circulation journal printed in French and sold by subscription under the masthead title of *Dialogue*. It does not have a broad audience, but its information is vital for the advancement of cancer healing. The *Dialogue* journal's editorial offices are located at the *Centre d'Innovations, de Recherches et d'Informations Scientifiques*, BP 36-38370 Saint-Prim, France. Tel. 04 74 56 58 00.

[5] The American College for Advancement in Medicine (ACAM) is a not-for-profit Organization dedicated to educating physicians and other health-care professionals on the safe and effective application of integrative medicine. ACAM's healthcare model focuses on prevention of illness and strives for total wellness. ACAM is the voice of integrative medicine; its goals are to improve physician skills, knowledge and diagnostic procedures as they relate to integrative medicine; to support integrative medicine research; and to provide education on current standards of care as well as additional approaches to patient care.

ACAM enables members of the public to connect with physicians who take an integrative approach to patient care and empowers individuals with information about integrative medicine treatment options. Celebrating more than a quarter century of service, ACAM represents over 1,500 physicians in thirty countries. ACAM is the largest and oldest organization of its kind in the world dedicated exclusively to serving the needs of the integrative medicine industry. * **For a full listing of all ACAM conventions, please visit www.acamnet.org.**

*Integrative medicine combines conventional care with alternative medicine to improve patient care. Rather than practice one type of medicine, integrative physicians will often combine therapies and treatment approaches to ensure the best results for their patients. ACAM physicians do not shun western medicine, in fact they practice western care every day. ACAM physicians are unique in that they incorporate *appropriate* and proven alternative treatment options.

[6] I possess a recorded interview that confirms Le Perlier's story. It is of the French licensed physician, P. K, M.D., of Versailles who was contacted by Mitterrand through one Mme. Pinjon. Mitterrand's official doctors, Drs. Gubler, Tareau, and Debré were not happy to share their patient with a newcomer. Dr. K. confirmed the efficacy of Dr. Beljanski's botanicals for the control of prostate cancer not only for Mitterrand but also for many of his other male patients. To gain his information on audiotape, I sat with Dr. P. K and his wife at dinner in a swank Paris

restaurant. The politically active physician spoke cautiously, haltingly, and with thought-filled projected intervals between statements. Getting definitive information from him was like pulling teeth, but I did receive some viable tidbits which confirmed his successful application of Beljanski's botanicals, including the administration of them to President François Mitterrand. This same physician provided me with a patient history of an eight-year-old boy for whom he reversed aplastic anemia (greatly reduced quantities of all blood cells lines) by use of Beljanski's therapies. With help from Dr. Beljanski's supplements, Dr. K. also caused the large-sized mediastinum (chest cavity) lymphoma tumor of a middle-age man to disappear in three weeks. This result occurred after radiotherapy had failed to give any positive response. It was a miracle, the Versailles physician said. Furthermore, Dr. P. K. told me more about his therapeutic achievements. They included the elimination of cancers of the breast and thymus by having his patients closely follow Dr. Beljanski's therapeutic recommendations.

[7] Causse, J.E.; Nawrocki, T.; Beljanski, M. "Human skin fibrosis RNase search for a biological inhibitor-regulator." *Deutsche Zeitschrift fur Onkologie* 23(5):137-139, 1994.

Notes to Chapter 1

[8] Gros, F.; Beljanski, M.; Macheboeuf, M.; Grumbach, F. "Comparaison biochimique d'une souche bacterienne sensible à la streptomycine avec une souche résistante de même espèce." *C.R. Acad. Sci.* 230:875-877, 1950.

Gros. F.; Beljanski, M.; Macheboeuf, M. "Mode d'action de la pénicilline chez *Staphylococcus aureus* inhibition d'un système enzymatique edtrait des bactéries." *C.R. Acad. Sci.* 231:184-186, 1950.

Gros. F.; Beljanski, M.; Macheboeuf, M. "Action de la pénicilline sur le métabolisme de la pénicilline sur le métabolisme de l'acide ribonucléique chez S*taphylococcus aureus.*" *Bull. Soc. Chim Biol.* 33:1696-1717,1951.

Gros, F.; Beljanski, M.; Macheboeuf, M.; Grumbach, F.; Boyer, F. "Activie biologique des combinaisons streptomycine-acides gras." *C.R. Acad. Sci.* 232:764-766, 1951.

Beljanski, M. "Etude de souches bactériennes résistantes a des antibiotiques. Comparaison avec des souches sensibles de mêmes eseces." *Ann. Biol.* 27:77-780, 1951.

Beljanski, M. "Etude des souches bactériennes résistantes a des antibiotiques. Comparaison avec des souches sensibles de mêmes eseces." These de Doctorates Sciences d'Etat, Université Parisla Sorbonne, 1951, Paris, Librairie Arnette, 1952.

Beljanski, M. "Action de la cocarboxylase sur le métabolisme des acides nucléiques chez *Staphylococcus aureus* sensible et résistant à la streptomycine." 2eme Congres Intern. De Biochimie, Paris, 1952. Resume des communications, 99.

Beljanski, M. "Comparaison de souches bactériennes résistantes a des antibiotiques avec des souches sensibles de même espece-I: Cas de la streptomycine." *Ann. Inst. Pasteur.* 83:80-101, 1952.

Beljanski, M. "Comparaison de souches bactériennes résistantes a des antibiotiques avec des souches sensibles de même espece-II: Cas de la pénicilline." *Ann. Inst. Pasteur.* 84:402-408, 1953.

Beljanski, M. "Comparaison de souches bactériennes résistantes a des antibiotiques avec des souches sensibles de même espèce-III: Cas du sulfamide-IV: Cas de l'azoture de sodium" *Ann. Inst. Pasteur.* 84:756-764, 1953.

Beljanski, M. "Comparaison de souches bactériennes résistantes à la streptomycine avec des souches sensibles de même espèce." *C.R. Acad. Sci.*, 236: 1102-1104, 1953.

Beljanski, M. & Gurmbach, F. "Etude biochimique d'une souche de Mycobacterium tuberculosis streptomycino-sensible et d'une souche streptomycino-resistante derive de la souche sensible." *C.R. Acad. Sci.*, 236:2111-2113, 1953.

Beljanski, M. "Etude des acides nucléiques de souches bactériennes résistantes à la streptomycine et de souches de mêmes espèces mais sensibles à l'antibiotiques." *Ann. Inst. Pasteur,* 85:463-469, 1953.

Beljanski, M. & Guelfi, J. "Etude a l'aide du 32P de l'accumulation des acides nucléiques chez *Staphylococcus aureus et Salmonella enteritidis* resistants et sensibles à la streptomycine." *Ann. Inst. Pasteur.,* 86:115-117, 1954.

Beljanski, M. "L'absence de cytochromes et de certains systèmes enzymatiques dans un noubeau mutant d'Escerichia coli streptomy-cino-resistant. Comparaison avec la souche sensible don't il derive." *C.R. Acad. Sci.,* 238:852-854, 1954.

Beljanski, M. "L'action de la ribonuclease et de la desoxyribonuclease sur l'incorporation de glycocolle radioacatif dans les proteins de lysats de *Micrococcus lysodeikticus.*" *Biochim Biophys. Acta.* 15:425-431, 1954.

Beljanski, M. "Isolement de mutants d'*Escherichia coli* streptomy-cino-resistants depourvus d'enzymes respiratoires. Action de l'hemine sur la formation de ces enzymes chez le mutant H-7." *C.R. Acad. Sci.,* 240:374-376, 1955.

Beljanski, M. "Formation d'enzymes respiratoires chez un mutant d'*Escherichia coli* streptomycino-resistant ne manifestant pas d'activite' respiratoire." 3eme Congres Intern. Biochim, Bruxelles. 1955, p.98 – Resumes des communications.

Latarjet, R. & Beljanski, M. "Photo-restoration in porphyrin-less mutants of *Escherichia coli.*" *Microbial Genetic Bulletin*, E. Witkins, 1955 – Resumes.

Beljanski, M. & Beljanski, M.S. "sur la formation d'enzymes respiratoires chez un mutant d'*Escherichia coli* strepomycino-resistant et auxotrophic pour l'hemine." *Ann. Inst. Pasteur.,* 922:396-412, 1957.

[9] Gros, F.; Beljanski, M.; Macheboeuf, M.; Grumbach, F. "Comparai-son biochimique d'une souche bacterienne sensible à la streptomycine avec une souche résistante de même espèce." *C.R. Acad. Sci.* 230:875-877, 1950.

Gros. F.; Beljanski, M.; Macheboeuf, M. "Mode d'action de la pénicilline chez Staphylococcus aureus inhibition d'un système enzymatique edtrait des bactéries." *C.R. Acad. Sci.* 231:184-186, 1950.

Gros. F.; Beljanski, M.; Macheboeuf, M. "Action de la pénicilline sur le métabolisme de la pénicilline sur le métabolisme de l'acide ribonucléique chez *Staphylococcus aureus.*" *Bull. Soc. Chim Biol.* 33:1696-1717,1951.

Gros, F.; Beljanski, M.; Macheboeuf, M.; Grumbach, F.; Boyer, F. "Activie biologique des combinaisons streptomycine-acides gras." *C.R. Acad. Sci.* 232:764-766, 1951.

[10] Beljanski, M. & Ochoa, S. "Protein biosynthesis by a cell-free bacterial system." *Proc. Nat. Acad. Sci., Biochemistry* 44:494-500, 1958.

Beljanski, M. & Ochoa, S. "Protein biosynthesis by a cell-free bacterial system." IVeme Congres Intern. Biochim., Vienne, 1958, p. 49 – Resumes des communications.

Beljanski, M. & Ochoa, S. "Protein biosynthesis by a cell-free bacterial system II-Further studies on the amino acid incorporation enzyme." *Proc. Nat. Acad. Sci.* 44:1157-1161, 1958.

Notes to Chapter 2

[11] "Antibiotics 1928 – 2000.) Millennium Bugs. http://www.abc.net.au/science/slab/antibiotics/history.htm. Access April 15, 2011. © 1999 Australian Broadcasting Corporation.

[12] *Ibid. Nature,* Watson, J.D. & Crick., F.H.

[13] Watson, J.D. *The Double Helix.* (New York: Atheneum, 1968).

[14] Starr, Barry. "DNA Mutations Cause Cancer: Cancer Runs in Families When Children Inherit a Premade Mutation | Suite101.com http://www.suite101.com/content/dna-mutations-cause-cancer-a44020#ixzz1NOARd0SK. Feb 8, 2008. May 24, 2011.

[15] Hall, John. "Destabilization of the DNA double helix in cancer. Mirko Beljanski's theory of carcinogenesis and anti-cancer extracts." *Townsend Letter for Doctors and Patients,* June, 2004.

findarticlesl.com/p/articles/mi_moisw/is_251/ai_n6167162/p8_21. April 14, 2011.

[16] Darnell, J.; Lodish, H.; Baltimore, D. *Molecular Biology*. (New York: Scientific American Books, 1998).

Meselson, M. & Stahl, F.V. "The replication of DNA." Cold Spring Harb. Symp. *Quant. Biol.* 23:9-12, 1958.

Mzibri, M. et al. "The Salmonella sulA-test: a new *in vitro* system to detect gerotoxins." *Mutat. Res.* 12, 369(3-4):195-208, 1996.

Schmid. W. "The micronucleus test." *Mutat. Res.* 31:9-15, 1995.

Notes to Chapter 3

[17] Hall, John. "Destabilization of the DAN double helix in cancer (get full citation from chapter 2)

[18] Beljanski, M. *The Regulation of DNA Replication and Transcription.* (New York: EVI Liberty Corp, 2003).

[19] Weinberg, Robert A. *One Renegade Cell: How Cancer Begins* (Science Master Series). New York: Basic Books, 1999.

[20] Ames, B.N.; Durston, W.E.; Yamasaki, E.; Lee, F.D. "Carcinogens are mutagens: a simple test system combining liver homogenates for activation and bacteria for detection." *Proc. Natn. Acad. Sci.* USA 70: 2281-2285 (1973).

[21] Beljanski, M.; Nawrocki, T.; LeGoff, L. "Possible role of markers synthesized during cancer evolution: I-Markers in mammalian tissues." *IRCS Med. Sci.*, 14: 809-810, 1979.

[22] These (A) and (B) phenomena have been observed by other biological scientists in multiple specialties as well; Beljanski clearly names these scientists in his 1983 book, cited in note 22.

[23] Le Goff, L. & Beljanski, M. "Cancer/anticancer dual action drugs in crown-gall tumors." IRCS Medical Science, 7:475, 1979.

Beljanski, M.; Le Goff, L.; Beljanski, M.S. "In vitro screening of carcinogens using DNA of the His-Mutant of *Salmonella typhimurium*." *Experimental Cellular Biology*, 50: 271-280, 1982.

Beljanski, M. & Le Goff, L. "Tumor promoter (TPA), DNA chain opening and unscheduled DNA synthesis." *IRCS Medical Science,* 11: 363-364, 1983.

[24] Saporto, Bill: "He Won His Battle with Cancer. So Why Are Millions of Americans still Losing Theirs?" *Time,* September 15, 2008, pp. 36-43.

[25] Doctor, K.S.; Reed, J.C., et al. "Cell deaths differ." *Apoptosis Database* 10(6):621-623, 2003.

Darnell, J.; Lodish, H.; Baltimore, D. *Molecular Biology.* (New York: Scientific American Books, 1998).

Meselson, M. & Stahl, F.V. "The replication of DNA." Cold Spring Harb. Symp. *Quant. Biol.* 23:9-12, 1958.

Mzibri, M., et al. "The Salmonella sulA-test: a new *in vitro* system to detect gerotoxins." *Mutat. Res.* 12, 369(3-4):195-208, 1996.

Schmid. W. "The micronucleus test." *Mutat. Res.* 31:9-15, 1995. Ames, B.; Less, F.; Durston, W. "An improved bacterial test system for the detection and classification of mutagens and carcinogens." *Proc. Natl. Acad. Sci.* USA, 70:782-786.

[26] A Variant of the Oncotest. If this variant aspect of the Oncotest isn't understandable, please do not worry. I have added it for the sake of sparking future research among oncologists into applying the Oncotest for its diagnostic and therapeutic effectiveness.

The principle of the Oncotest is that DNA of various origins can be selected for testing without the same limitations as in the Ames test. But Beljanski also found that the Oncotest helped to clarify the results of the Ames test.

DNA from the bacterial strains of Dr. Ames' were labeled in two ways: *His+ non-mutant strain* and Dr. Ames' labeled *His- mutant strain*; both could be used in order to screen molecules in the Oncotest. The result? No carcinogens escape identification as they all test positive in the Oncotest.

In fact, if we isolate and purify DNA from the His- mutants of the *salmonella typhimurium* organism, it is possible to do a follow up to the Oncotest. Each carcinogenic agent incubated in the presence of purified *His-* DNA-induced strand separation, stimulated DNA synthesis as efficiently as that observed with known chemical carcinogens. These observations suggest that negative results obtained in the Ames test with so many carcinogenic agents, using the bacteria *S. typhimurium*, in truth indicate a permeability barrier of bacteria. Mutant *His-* DNA *in vitro* reactivity with carcinogens/mutagens or non-mutagens, indicate that, for detection of carcinogens, purified DNA from *His-* mutants can be used in the Oncotest.

The perfect correlation between results obtained both in the Oncotest and this variant of the Oncotest using DNA from the bacterial mutants clearly explains to molecular biologists the mechanism of gene activation related in Mirko Beljanski's book and in his various publications. These same results were also obtained using healthy plant cell DNA and plant tumor.

NOTES TO CHAPTER 4

[27] "How many people die from cancer each year?" Nanomedicine-center.com. http://www.nanomedicinecenter.com/article/how-many-people-die-from-cancer-each-year/ Feb. 1, 2010. July 20, 2011.

[28] John Hall, Ph.D., corroborates Mme. Beljanski's findings by pointing out that it is now common knowledge among health professionals: "many chemotherapeutic drugs are themselves potent carcinogens." In "Destabilization of the DNA double helix in cancer: Mirko Beljanski's theory of carcinogenesis and anti-cancer extracts" (see note in chapter 2 and 3).

[29] *A Pioneer in Biomedicine*, pg. 72.

[30] *A Pioneer in Biomedicine*, pg. 72.

[31] Coles, L. Stephen, M.D., Ph.D. *Extraordinary Healing. How the Discoveries of Mirko Beljanski, the world's first green molecular*

biologist, can protect and restore your health. Topanga, CA: Freedom Press, 2011.

[32] Beljanski M., et al. "Differential susceptibility of cancer and normal DNA template allows the detection of carcinogens and anticancer drugs. Third NCI-EORTC symposium of new drug therapy." Bordet Institute, Brussels, 1981.

[33] *Molecular Biology & Biotechnology: A Comprehensive Desk Reference,* (Ed.) Robert A. Meyers, (New York City: VCH Publishing Co., 1995).

[34] Beljanski, M., Beljanski, M.S. Three alkaloids as selective destroyers of the proliferative capacity of cancer cells. *IRCS Med. Sci.* 1984. 12: pp. 587-588.

Beljanski, M., Bourgarel, P., Beljanski, M.S. Correlation between *in vitro* DNA Synthesis, DNA Strand Separation and *in vivo* Multiplication of Cancer Cells. *Expl. Cell. Biol.,* 1981. 49: pp. 220-231.

Beljanski, M., Crochet, S., Beljanski, M.S. PB100: A Potent and Selective Inhibitor of Human BCNU Resistant Glioblastoma Cell Multiplication. Anticancer Research, 1993. 13: pp. 2301-2308.

Beljanski, M., Crochet, S. Selective inhibitor (PB-100) of human glioblastoma cell multiplication. *Journal of Neuro-Oncology.* 1994. 21: p. 62.

Beljanski, M., Crochet, S. The selective anticancer agents PB-100 and BG-8 are active against human melanoma cells, but do not affect non-malignant fibroblasts. *International Journal of Oncology.* 1996. 8: 1143-1148.

[35] The original study is from Beljanski, M. "The anticancer agent PB-100, selectively active on malignant cells, inhibits multiplication of sixteen malignant cell lines, even multidrug resistant." *Genetics and Molecular Biology,* 23, 1, 29-33 (2000). In *Extraordinary Healing,* Stephen Coles has extracted the percentages from the material presented in Beljanski study, 73.

[36] Beljanski, M. & Le Goff, L. "Tumor promoter (TPA), DNA chain opening and unscheduled DNA synthesis". *IRCS Med. Sci.*, 11: 363-364, 1983.

Le Goff, L. & Beljanski, M. "The *in vivo* effects of opines and other compounds on DNAs originating from bacteria and from healthy and tumorous plant tissues." *Expl. Cell. Biol.* 53: 335-350, 1985.

Beljanski, M.; Le Goff, L.; Beljanski, M.S. "Differential susceptibility of cancer and normal DNA templates allows the detection of carcinogens and anticancer drugs." *Third NCI-EORTC Symp. On New Drugs in Cancer Therapy.* Institut Bordet, Bruxelles, 1981.

Le Goff, L. & Beljanski, M. "Crown-gall tumor stimulation or inhibition: correlation with DNA strand separation". *Proc. Fifth Int. Conf. on Plant Path. & Bact.* Cali. pp. 295-307, 1981.

Beljanski, M.; Le Goff, L.; Faivre-Amiot, A. "Preventive and curative anticancer drug. Application to crown-gall tumors." *Acta Horticulturae*, 125: 239-248, 1982.

Le Goff, L. & Beljanski, M. "Cancer/anti-cancer dual action drugs in crown-gall tumors." *IRCS Medical Science*, 7: 475, 1979.

In the Oncotest, we have seen that hormones destabilize DNA and therefore act as potential carcinogens. We find again that in plant cancers, hormonal action is necessary (as confirmed by numerous researchers) prior to the induction of cancer in plants. The Beljanski team had researched and developed these studies on cancer induction and inhibition in plants at length and showed, in particular, the essential role of plant hormones in this process. (See Beljanski's publications # 72, 81, 85, 90, 91, 93, 94, 97, 101, 102, 113 in Appendix C.)

[38] Beljanski, M.; Aaron-da-Cunha, Y.; Beljanski, M.S.; Manigual, P.; Bourgarel, P. "Isolation of the tumor-inducing RNA from oncogenic and non-oncogenic *Agrobacterium tumefaciens.*" *Proc. Nat. Acad. Sci.* (USA), 71: 1585-1589, 1974.

Le Goff, L.; Aaron-Da-Cunha, Y.; Beljanski, M. "RNA fraction from several non-oncogenic strains of *Agrobacterium tumefaciens* as tumor-inducing agent in Datura Stramonium". XIIth Intern. Bot. Congress. Resumes, Leningrad, 1975.

[39] J.L. Hall. Springer, D.L. Bemis. "A Novel combination of plant extracts with promising anti-prostate cancer activity." *Townsend Letter for Doctors and Patients,* Dec, 2004. Information taken from Beljanski study: Beljanski, M., Beljanski, M.S. Three alkaloids as selective destroyers of cancer cells in mice. Synergy with classic anticancer drugs. *Oncology,* 1986. 43: 198-203.

[40] *Extraordinary Healing,* 93-102.

[41] Debra Bemis, et al. "A Novel Plant Extract Containing Alkaloids in the B-Carboline Family with Promising Anti-Prostate Cancer Activity." Columbia University Medical Center College of Physicians and Surgeons. Abstract. Presented to the Society of Integrative Oncology, Nov. 17-19, 2004.

[42] Debra Bemis, et al. "β-Carboline Alkaloid-Enriched Extract from the Amazonian Rain forest Tree Pao Pereira Suppresses Prostate Cancer Cells." *Journal for the Society for Integrative Oncology,* Vol 7, no 2 (spring) 2009. 59-65.

[43] Burchill, Melissa. "Two Herbal Extracts for Protecting Prostate Cell DNA." *Integrative Medicine.* Vol. 9, no. 2, Apr/May 2010. 32-36.

[44] Debra Bemis et al. "B-Carboline Alkaloid –Enriched Extract from the Amazonian Rain Forest Re Pao Pereira Suppresses Prostate Cancer Cells." *Journal for the Society for Integrative Oncology,* Vol 7, no 2 (spring) 2009. 59-65.

[45] C.G. Nordau and M.S. Beljanski. *A Pioneer in Biomedicine: Concepts, Theories and Applications.* New York: Edition EVI Liberty Corp, 2000.

[46] Mercola, Joseph. www.Mercola.com.

[47] Epstein, Samual S. *The Politics of Cancer Revisited.* East Ridge Press, 1998.

48 Beljanski, M. "A new approach to cancer therapy." *Proceedings of the International Seminar: Traditional Medicine: a Challenge of the 21st Century, Calcutta* (Ed.) Biswapati Mukharjee, 7-9 Nov. 1992.

49 *The Merck Manual of Medical Information; Home Edition.* Berkow, R.; Beers, M.H.; Fletcher, A.J., Eds. (Whitehouse Station, New Jersey: Merck Research Laboratories, 1997), pp. 549-551.

50 Schachter, M.B. *The Natural Way to a Healthy Prostate.* (New Canaan, Connecticut: Keats Publishing, Inc., 1995), p. 6.

51 Walker, M. "The urologist with zero tolerance for prostate problems." *Townsend Letter for Doctors & Patients* 201:78-82, April 2001.

NOTES TO CHAPTER 5

52 http://ict.sagepub.com

53 http://www.holisticurology.columbia.edu/_aboutus/Mission.html. July 21, 2011.

54 Jonathan Weiner. "The Mind of a Disease." *New York Times Book Review.* Nov 12, 2010. (http://www.nytimes.com/2010/11/14/books/review/Weiner-t.html.)

55 Burchill, Melissa. "Two Herbal Extracts for Protecting Prostate Cell DNA." *Integrative Medicine.* Vol. 9, no. 2, Apr/May 2010. 36.

56 M. Beljanski, M.S. Beljanski. 'Three alkaloids as selective destroyers of cancer cells in mice. Synergy with classic anticancer drugs." *Onkologie,* 43, 1986, pp. 198-203.

Nordau C. G. and Monique Beljanski. *A Pioneer in Medicine: Concepts, Theories, Applications.* New York: EVI Liberty Corp, 2000.

57 *Extraordinary Healing,* pg. 41.

58 *A Pioneer in Biomedicine, chapter 3.*

59 Coles, L. Stephen. "RNA Fragments, Anti-Aging, and Immune Health" *The Doctors' Prescription for Healthy Living.* Sept. 2009.

60 MedicineNet.com. http://www.medterms.com/script/main/art.asp?articlekey=5367 May 5, 2011.

[61] BELJANSKI, M.; BELJANSKI, M. S.; PLAWECKI, M.; MANIGAULT, P. "ARN-fragments, amorceurs nécessaires à la réplication « in vitro » des ADN." *C.R. Acad. Sci.*, 280:363-366, 1975, (série D).

[62] BELJANSKI, M.; PLAWECKI, M.; BOURGAREL, P.; BELJANSKI, M.S. "Leucocyte recovery with short-chain RNA fragments in cyclophosphamide-treated rabbits." *Cancer Treatment Reports.* 67: 611-619, 1983.

[63] BELJANSKI, M.; PLAWECKI, M.; BOURGAREL, P.; BELJANSKI, M.S. "Nouvelles substances (R.L.B.) actives dans la leucopoïèse et la formation des plaquettes." Bull. Acad. Nat. Med., 162(6) :475-781, 1978.

BELJANSKI, M. & PLAWECKI, M. "Particular RNA fragments as promoters of leukocyte and platelet formations in rabbits". *Exp. Cell Biol.*, 1979, 47, pp. 218-225.

BELJANSKI, M. "Oligoribo-nucleotides, promoters of leucocyte and platelet genesis in animals depleted by anticancer drugs". NCI-EORTC *Symposium on nature, prevention and treatment of clinical toxicity of anticancer agents.* Institut Bordet, Bruxelles, 1980.

BELJANSKI, M.; PLAWECKI, M.; BOURGAREL, P.; BELJANSKI, M.S. "Short chain RNA fragments as promoters of leucocyte and platelet genesis in animals depleted by anti-cancer drugs". In *The Role of RNA in Development and Reproduction.* Sec. Int. Symposium, M.C. Niu and H.H. Chuang Eds Van Nostrand Reinhold Company. (Beijing: Science Press, April 25-30, 1980), pp.79-113.

PLAWECKI, M. & BELJANSKI, M. "Comparative study of *Escherichia coli* endotoxin. Hydrocortisone and Beljanski leucocyte restorer activity in cyclophosphamide-treated rabbits." *Proc. of the Soc. for Exp. Biol. and Med.*, 168: 408-413, 1981.

DONADIO, D.; LORHO, R.; CAUSSE, J.E.; NAWROCKI, T.; BELJANSKI, M. "RNA fragments (RLB) and tolerance of cytostatic treatments in hematology: A preliminary study about two non-Hodgkin malignant lymphoma cases." *Deutsche Zeitschrift für Onkologie*, 23(2): 33-35, 1991. (OLD NOTE 39-43)

[64] Schachter, Michael, M.D., CNS. "Integrative Oncology for Clinicians and Cancer Patients." From an expanded lecture presented at the International Society of Integrative Medicine meeting in Tokyo, Japan on July 19, 2009. From http://www.breastcancerchoices.org/files/Schachter_PDF_File_from_ICIM_Journal.pdf.

[65] Robert D. Levin, MaryAnn Daehler, James F. Grutsch, John L. Hall, Dignant Gupta, Christopher G. Lis. "Dose escalation study of anti-thrombocytopenic agent in patients with chemotherapy induced thrombocytopenia." BMC Cancer 2010, 10:565. http://www.biomedcentral.com/1471-2407/10/565.

[66] L. Stephen Coles, M.D., Ph.D. "RNA Fragments, Anti-aging Medicine and Immune Health." *The Doctors' Prescription for Healthy Living.* September, 2009. pg. 25-26.

[67] John W. Gofman, MD, Ph.D. "Radiation from Medical Procedures in the Pathogenesis of Cancer and Ischemic Heart Disease: Dose-Response Studies with Physicians per 100,000 Population" San Francisco: Committee for Nuclear Responsibility, Inc., 1999.

[68] Kaplan. Adv. Dermatol. 2: 19-46, 1987.

[69] *Extraordinary Healing*, 53-55.

[70] Soloman, P.R.; Adams, F., et al. "*Ginkgo* for memory enhancement: a randomized controlled trial." *JAMA* 288 (7):835-840, 2002.

Burns, N.R.; Bryan, J.; Nettelbeck, T. "*Ginkgo biloba*: no robust effect on cognitive abilities or mood in healthy, young or older adults." *Hum. Psycho. Pharmacol.* Dec. 2005.

Clostre, F. "*Ginkgo biloba* extract. State of knowledge in the dawn of the year 2000." *Ann. Pharm.* Fr. 57 Suppl. 1:158-188, 1990.

[71] Rosen, I.; Fischer, T., et al. "Correlation between lung fibrosis and radiation therapy dose after concurrent radiation therapy and chemotherapy for limited small cell lung cancer." *Radiology*; 221:614, 2001.

[72] Saflotti, V.; Shubik, R. "The role of burning in carcinogenesis." *Br. J. Cancer,* 10:54-57, 1956.

Sirsat, M.V. & Shrikhande, S.S. "Histochemical studies on squamous cell carcinomas of the skin arising in burn scars with special reference to histogenesis." *Indian J. Cancer* 3:157-169, 1967.

Beljanski, M. "Radioprotection of irradiated; mice-mechanisms and synergistic action of WR-2721 and R.L.B." *Deutsche Zeitschrift ur Onkologie*, 23(6): 155-159, 1991.

[73] Natural Source International, the company who manufactures the Beljanski products, in conjunction with CIRIS, conducted the survey, tabulated the results, and shared the information in their newsletter.

[74] Beljanski, M. "Radioprotection of irradiated; mice-mechanisms and synergistic action of WR-2721 and R.L.B." *Deutsche Zeitschrift ur Onkologie*, 23(6): 155-159, 1991.

Causse, J.E.; Nawrocki, T.; Beljanski, M. "Human skin fibrosis RNase search for a biological inhibitor-regulator": -*Deut. Zeit. Fur Onk.*, 26, 5, 1994, pp. 137-139.

Nordau, C.G. & Beljanski, M. *A Pioneer in Biomedicine,* (New York: EVI Liberty Corp., 2003), pp. 66, 116, 122.

[75] Le Goff, L. & Beljanski, M. "Cancer/anticancer dual action drugs in crown- gall tumors." *IRCS Medical Science,* 7:475, 1979.

Beljanski, M.; Le Goff, L.; Beljanski, M.S. "In vitro screening of carcinogens using DNA of the His-Mutant of *Salmonella typhimurium.*" Experimental Cellular Biology, 50: 271-280, 1982.

Beljanski, M. & Le Goff, L. "Tumor promoter (TPA), DNA chain opening and unscheduled DNA synthesis." *IRCS Medical Science,* 11: 363-364, 1983.

[76] Hoffmann, D. *The Complete Illustrated Holistic Herbal: a Safe and Practical Guide to Making and Using Herbal Remedies.* (New York: Barnes and Noble Books, 1996), P. 101.

NOTES TO CHAPTER 6

[77] Le Perlier, J.P. *Enguete Sur un Survivant Illegal.* (Paris: Ed. Guy Tredaniel Publishing Co., 2002).

[78] Temin, H.M. "Mechanism of cell transformation by RNA tumor viruses." *A. Rev. Microbiol.* 25:609-648, 1971.

[79] Beljanski, M. "Synthese *in vitro* de l'AND sur une matrice d'ARN par une transcriptase d'*Escharichia coli.*" *C.R. Acad. Sci.* 274:2801-2804 (serie D), 1972.

[80] Beljanski, M. "Separation de la transcriptase inverse de l'AND polymerase AND dependante. Analyse de l'AND synthetise sur le modele de l'ARN transformant." *C.R.Acad. Sci.* 276:1625-1628, 193.

Beljanski, M. & Beljanski, M.S. "RNA-bound reverse transcriptase in Escherichia coli and in vitro synthesis of a complementary DNA." *Biochemical genetics*, 12:163-180, 1974.

[81] Donadio D., et al. "Tolerance and feasibility of a 12-month therapy using the antiretroviral agent PB-100 in AIDS-related complex patients." *Dtsch. Zschr. Onkol.* 26(6):145-149, 1994.

The published results indicate the following significant information for patients with severe HIV infections:

1) no drug resistance was developed;
2) the CD4+ count in infected HIV blood improved instead of continuing to fall;
3) the CD4/CD8 ratio increased and was thus improved.

Looking at number three above, see that a different alteration occurred: The sick patients' P24 antigen, a highly significant measure of immunity read by infectious disease specialists, did not change in eight of the HIV patients; in two others, however, the same antigen became negative in one patient and stable in another. Thus we see a tendency toward normality by 50 percent.

[82] Nordau, G.C. & Beljanski, M.S. *A Pioneer in Biomedicine.* (New York: EVI Liberty Corp., 2003).

[83] http://www.avert.org/aids-funding.htm. "Funding for the AIDS and HIV epidemic." May 5, 2011.

[84] http://www.cancer.gov/cancertopics/factsheet/NCI/research-funding.

NOTES TO CHAPTER 7

[85] "Sticker shock a side effect of cancer remedies." Cancer on MSNBC.com. http://www.msnbc.msn.com/id/23783216/ns/health-cancer/t/sticker-shock-side-effect-cancer-remedies/. April 18, 2011.

[86] Hoffman, D. *The Complete Illustrated Holistic Herbal: A Safe and Practical Guide to Making and Using Herbal Remedies.* (New York: Barnes and Noble Books, 1996), p. 10.

[87] Murray, M.T. & Pizzorno, J.E. *Encyclopedia of Natural Medicine.* (Rocklin, California: Prima Publishing, 1991), pp. 6 & 7.

[88] "$34 billion spent yearly on alternative medicine." MSNBC.com. http://www.msnbc.msn.com/id/32219873/ns/health-alternative_medicine/t/billion-spent-yearly-alternative-medicine/.

[89] Werbach, M.R. & Murray, M.T. *Botanical Influences on Illness: A Sourcebook of Clinical Research.* (Tarzana, California: Third Line Press, 1994), p. 2.

[90] *The Complete German Commission E Monographs: Therapeutic Guide to Herbal Medicies.* Austin, TX: The American Botanical Council, 1999.

[91] Werbach, M.R. & Murray, M.T. *Botanical Influences on Illness: A Sourcebook of Clinical Research.* (Tarzana, California: Third Line Press, 1994), p. 2.

Keller, K. "Legal requirements for the use of phytopharmaceutical drugs in the Federal Republic of Germany." *J. Ethnopharmacal* 32:225-229, 1991.

[92] Beljanski, M. & Crochet, S. "The anticancer agent PB-100 concentrates in the nucleus and nucleoli of human glioblastoma cells but does not enter normal astrocytes." *International Journal of Oncology* 7 (1995): 81-85.

Beljanski, M. & Crochet, S. "The selective anticancer agents PB-100 and BG-8 are active against human melanoma cells, but do not affect nonmalignant fibroblasts." *International Journal of Oncology* 8 (1996): 1143-1148.

Beljanski, M. "The anticancer agent PB-100, selectively active on malignant cells, inhibits multiplication of sixteen malignant cell lines, even multi-drug resistant." *Genet. Mol. Biol.* 23:1 (2000).

[93] Beljanski, M., et al. "Leukocyte recovery with short-chain RNA fragments in cyclophosphamide-treated rabbits." *Cancer Treatment Reports* 67 (1983): 611-619.

Donadio, D., et al. "RNA fragments (RLB) and tolerance of cytostatic treatments in hematology: A preliminary study about two non-Hodgkin malignant lymphoma cases." *Deutsche Zeitschrift für Onkologie* 23:2 (1991): 33-35.

[94] Nordau, G.C. & M.S. Beljanski. *A Pioneer in Biomedicine.* New York: Evi Liberty Corp., 2003.

Caussé et al. "Human skin fibrosis RNase search for a biological inhibitor-regulator." *Deutsche Zeitschrift für Onkologie* 26:5 (1994): 137-139.

[95] Douglas Kalman, Ph.D., MS, RD, CCRC, FACN. "Research Process: Are RCTs the Wave of the Future: If so, there as some basic things your company should know about study design. http://www.nutraceuticalsworld.com/issues/2011-04/view_columns/research-process-are-rcts-the-wave-of-the-future-/. April 2011. August 16, 2011.

See also, "The End of Supplements in America?" editorial. http://www.life-enhancement.com/article_template.asp?ID=2422. 2011. August 16, 2011.

NOTES FOR CHAPTER 8

[96] *Extraordinary Healing,* chapters six and seven.

[97] Marcowith, C. "Beljanski application." In *Cancer: The Beljanski Approach.* (New York City: EVI Liberty Corporation, 2003).

[98] Gerson, C. & Walker, M. *The Gerson Therapy: The Amazing Nutritional Program for Cancer and Other Illness* (New York City: Kensington Publishing Corp., 2001).

[99] Beljanski, M.S. *Chronique d'une 'fatwa' Scientifique.* (Paris : Tredaniel, 2003).

NOTES TO CHAPTER 9

[100] *Extraordinary Healing*, 84.

[101] *Extraordinary Healing*, 81.

[102] *Extraordinary Healing*, 82.

[103] *Extraordinary Healing*, chapter 7.

[104] *Extraordinary Healing*, 86.

[105] *Extraordinary Healing*, 86.

[106] *Extraordinary Healing*, 88.

[107] Spiegelman, S. "An approach to the experimental analysis of precellular evolution." *Quart.Rev.Biophys.*, 4: 213-253, 1971.

[108] Schrodinger, E. *What Is Life?* (Boston: Cambridge University Press. Reprint Ed. Jan. 31, 1992.) ISBN : 0521427088.

[109] De Duve, Christian. *Blueprint for a Cell: The Nature and Origin of Life*. Burlington N.C.: The Carolina Biological Supply Company, 1991.

[110] *Extraordinary Healing*, 89.

[111] *Extraordinary Healing*, 89.

Appendix A
Resource Guide

For information on Dr. Mirko Beljanski and his products:

The Beljanski Foundation
> The Beljanski Foundation
> 5 Tudor City Place # 2209
> New York, NY 10017
> Tel: 646-808-5583
> Fax: 212-308-7014
> info@beljanskifoundation.com
> www.Beljanski.com

CIRIS: *Centre d'Innovations, de Recherches et d'Informations Scientifiques* (Center of Scientific Innovations, Research, and Information)
> Association CIRIS
> BP 9
> 17550-Dolus d'Oléron, France
> Phone : 05.46.75.39.75 (For Voicemail Only)
> 04.74.56.58.00
> Fax : 05.46.75.39.75
> Email : info@beljanski.com
> Communication in French only.

For English-speaking persons who want to know more about CIRIS, please contact the Beljanski Foundation at the phone numbers listed above.

Physicians who practice CAIM (Complimentary, Alternative, and Integrative Medicine)

Please visit the **American College for the Advancement in Medicine (ACAM):**

Website: www.ACAM.org.

Author's Note: The list of United States holistic physicians on the ACAM site receives updating twice yearly. For the most current information you may wish to contact ACAM's Director of Communications, Sharon Urch. You can reach Ms. Urch by telephoning (949) 309-3520 or FAX her at (949) 309-3538; or write to the American College for Advancement in Medicine, 24411 Ridge Route, Suite 115, Laguna Hills, California 92653; Email: executivedirector@acam.org.

Physicians Cited in the Text:

Health Professional Michael B. Schachter, M.D.

Although Board Certified in Psychiatry, holistic physician Michael B. Schachter, M.D., Medical Director of the Schachter Center for Complementary Medicine in Suffern, New York, utilizes treatment methods of CAIM in his active antimalignancy practice. Dr. Schachter was President of the American College for Advancement in Medicine during the years 1989 through 1991. In lectures and published journal articles, he has reported extensively on the discoveries of Mirko Beljanski, Ph.D. You may read some of his presentations on Beljanski by bringing up his several websites at www.schachtercenter.com/mirko_beljanski1.htm or www.mbschachter.com or www.schachtercenter.com.

The Schachter Center for Complementary Medicine is located at Two Executive Boulevard, Suite 202, Suffern, New York 10901 USA; telephone (845) 368-4700; FAX (845) 368-4727; Dr. Michael Schachter's personal Email is mbschachter@optonline.net.

Health Professional Ronald E. Wheeler, M.D.

An interventional urologist specializing in pathology of the prostate, Ronald E. Wheeler, M.D., is Medical Director of the Diagnostic Center for Disease, formerly known as the Prostatitis & Prostate Cancer Center of Sarasota, Florida. Dr. Wheeler utilizes unique methods of diagnosis and prudent dietary adjustments for improving his patients' prostate health, lowering their prostate cancer risk. He has combined particular natural herbal and nutritional ingredients plus certain minerals, vitamins, antioxidants and amino acids in a capsule. This self-administered encapsulated remedy that he calls PEENUTS® is an acronym for Power to Empty Every time while Never Urinating Too Soon.

The Wheeler Diagnostic Center for Disease is located at 1250 South Tamiami Trail, Suite One North, Sarasota, Florida 34239 USA; telephone (877) 766-8400 or (941) 957-0007; telefax (941) 957-1033; Dr. Ronald E. Wheeler's personal Email is prostadoc@aol.com; The Center website is www.theprostatecenter.com; also see Dr. Ronald Wheeler's adjunctive website at www.mrisusa.com; the PEENUTS telephone is (888) 733-6887; the PEENUTS website is www.peenuts.com.

Homeopath Leonard Haimes, M.D.
Nutritionist, Holistic Physician and Chelation Therapist

Practicing holistic medicine for over fifty years with specialties in chelation therapy and homeopathy, Leonard Haimes, M.D. is much loved and respected by his vast number of patients, friends, and other well-wishers. He has preserved lives, limbs, and longevity for upwards of no less than sixty-thousand people. Dr. Haimes eliminates their requirement for any hospitalization simply by keeping them in optimal health, and he does this without resorting to the use of laboratory-derived drugs.

Specialty health problems which are successfully treated by Dr. Leonard Haimes include erectile dysfunction, premature ejaculation, balancing for bio-identical hormones, sexual organ rejuvenation, general sexual enhancement, weight management, immune system improvement, allergy system rejuvenation, human growth hormone enhancement, pain management, and correction for environmental & internal medicine dysfunction.

The Haimes Centre Clinic had been directed by Leonard Haimes, M.D. but Dr. Haimes closed its doors during the second month of 2011. His patients miss him.

The Gonzalez/Kelly Therapy

Pancreatic enzyme therapy first utilized against all kinds of cancers by the non-conventionally practicing biological dentist William Donald Kelly, D.D.S., has shown remarkable success as a non-invasive and non-pharmaceutical healing technique. CAIM oncologist Nicholas J. Gonzalez, M.D., conducted a double-blind, placebo-controlled study and treatment trial on enzymatic applications for pancreatic cancer. He had studied under the now deceased Dr. Wm. D. Kelly, and today Dr. Gonzalez uses proteolytic enzymes extracted from the organs of New Zealand lambs. His investigations are carrying the Kelly method much further than the originator had gone. Dr. Gonzalez exclusively administers to patients affected by malignancies of the pancreas; for this condition he uses only proteolytic enzymes and does not permit any other therapies, including Beljanski's botanicals and RNA fragments. In fact, he is experiencing a relatively high rate of success in causing pancreatic cancer remission by his application of proteolytic enzyme therapy.

The Gonzalez NCI study group is now filled with trial recipients so that no more patients are being accepted at this time. However, people may receive more information about the proteolytic enzymes derived from the animal pancreas by contacting the offices of Dr. Nicholas Gonzalez at 36 East 36th Street, Suite 204, New York, New York 10016 USA; telephone (212) 213-3337; telefax (212) 213-3414.

The Gerson Therapy

Another holistic dietary, detoxifying, and nutritional supplement program that shows success for the treatment of nearly all cancers is the Gerson Therapy that had been developed by Max Gerson, M.D. It is such a stringent and disciplined treatment that someone achieving success with this program requires a strong will to live as the motive for accomplishing it.

The Gerson Therapy incorporates a daily drinking of large amounts of carrot, apple, and green juices. Additionally, The Gerson Therapy necessitates another somewhat unusual practice, the instilling of multiple daily coffee enemas for detoxification of the liver and other organs. The program's five required coffee enemas a day tend to pull out the accumulated cellular poisons produced by cancer cell pathology.

It's acknowledged by most CAIM health professionals that the Gerson Program recommended by Charlotte Gerson, daughter of the program's developer, has saved more people from dying of numerous types of malignancies than any other therapy in the health-care profession today.

Charlotte Gerson is founder of an excellent and highly respected cancer correction information and treatment source, The Gerson Institute. Dr. Morton Walker and Charlotte Gerson co-authored a detailed text about the Gerson treatmen program, *The Gerson Therapy.*

You may contact the organization's executive director, Anita Wilson, located at 1572 Second Avenue, San Diego, California 92101 USA. The Gerson Institute's international telephone for the U.S.A. and Canada may be found at (800) 838-2256 or for the U.S.A. only telephone to (888) 443-7766 or (619) 685-5353; FAX (619) 685-5363, website is www.gerson.org or www.gersonmiracle.org.

Health Professional Associations with Members Who Utilize Dr. Beljanski's Products:

American Association of Naturopathic Physicians (AANP)

This health professional organization, the AANP, provides a listing of American doctors of naturopathy (N.D.s) who administer natural and non-toxic therapies. Contact the AANP by telephone at (703) 556-9728; website is www.naturopathic.org.

American Holistic Medical Association (AHMA)

This health professional organization, the AHMA, provides a list of holistic medical doctors who employ complementary, alternative, integrative medicine (CAIM); telephone (703) 556-9728; website is www.holisticmedicine.org.

CancerHelp®

CancerHelp®, a registered comprehensive cancer information source for all inquirers, is maintained by the CancerHelp Institute, 1000 Skokie Boulevard, Suite 100, Wilmette, Illinois 60091 USA; telephone (847) 256-3093; telefax (847) 256-4985; Email is info@cancerhelpinstitute.org; website is www.cancerhelp.org.

National Foundation for Alternative Medicine (NFAM)

The NFAM has evaluated 67 holistic healthcare clinics in 20 countries and is developing a composite picture of how cancer patients are treated worldwide, especially throughout Europe and the United States. You may contact the NFAM by telephoning (202) 463-4900; website is www.nfam.org.

National Center for Complementary and Alternative Medicine (NCCA)

The NCCA provides the means to find journal citations related to complementary, alternative, and integrative medicine on the United States National Library of Medicine database; telephone (888) 644-6226; two websites exist for the NCCA which are www.nlm.nih.gov and/or www.nccam/camonpubmed.html.

The Natural Pharmacist

This organization provides a searchable database of vitamin, mineral, and herbal monographs, including Dr. Beljanski's supplements. Its monographs describe the latest research, caveats, and cautions connected with immune system boosting therapies; telephone (800) 637-7784; website is www.tnp.com.

Center for Holistic Urology

At the Columbia University College of Physicians and Surgeons, Associate Research Scientist Debra L. Bemis, Ph.D., and Research Urologist Aaron Katz, M.D., both participate in the Center of Holistic Urology in the University's Department of Urology at New York Presbyterian Hospital; 161 Fort Washington Avenue, New York, New York 10032 USA; telephone (212) 305-5727; telefax (212) 305-1564; the Center's website is www.holisticurology.com; its Email is dlb2004@columbia.edu.

Hyperbaric Services of the Palm Beaches, LLC

Hyperbaric oxygen therapy (HBOT) is available around the world for its safe, non-invasive, and fast-healing ability to bathe a person's entire body in the nutrient of life: oxygen. Cancer cells cannot exist when bathed in an oxygen environment. For instance, in the State of Florida, Hyperbaric Services of the Palm Beaches, LLC, offers oxygen's vital cellular nourishment in private, single-body Sechrist Industry 3600 monoplace oxygen therapy chambers in a beautifully appointed, new facility. Patients find the therapy experience comfortable, relaxing, and even recreational from the personal entertainment center offered including a television and DVD.

The compassionate and experienced staff at Hyperbaric Services of the Palm Beaches, LLC is committed to working closely with you and your physician to improve one's quality of life wanted by use of HBOT. Each staff member is Hyperbaric certified, including three staff physicians trained in Hyperbaric Oxygen Medicine. This facility is special because it is the only Joint Commission on Accreditation of Health Organizations (JCAHO) freestanding hyperbaric facility in the United States.

Under the administrative direction of Constance Governale, this HBOT facility is located on the grounds of the Delray Medical Center at 5130 Linton Boulevard, Suite H3 & H4, Delray Beach, FL 33484; telephone (800) 983-8582 or (561) 819-6125; telefax (561) 819-6127; inquire via Email: oxygen4u@bellsouth.net or learn lots more at the facility's website: www.palmbeachhyperbaric.com.

Dr. Morton Walker co-authored what is considered the definitive health-consumer text on oxygen treatment with the now deceased Richard Neubaurer, M.D.: *Hyperbaric Oxygen Therapy.*

For a complete bibliography of Dr. Walker's ninety-two published works, please refer to www.DrMortonWalker.com.

Appendix B
Scientific Publications of Mirko Beljanski, Ph.D.

The following lists all of the scientific publications produced by Dr. Mirko Beljanski. They are presented in chronological order and many of them are in French as that is the language in which they were published. No attempt has been made by the publisher to translate the material.

1. - A propos du microdosage du ribose dans les acides nucléiques et leurs dérivés:
   a) M. BELJANSKI, M. MACHEBOEUF, C.R. Soc. Biol. 1949, CXLIII, pp.174-175.
   b) M. BELJANSKI, Ann. Inst. Pasteur, 1949, 76, pp. 451-455.

2. - F. GROS, M. BELJANSKI, M. MACHEBOEUF, F. GRUMBACH, «Comparaison biochimique d'une souche bactérienne sensible à la streptomycine avec une souche résistance de même espèce». C.R. Acad. Sci., 1950, 230, pp. 875-877.

3. - F. GROS, M. BELJANSKI, M. MACHEBOEUF, «Mode d'action de la pénicilline chez Staphylococcus aureus. Inhibition d'un système enzymatique extrait des bactéries ». C.R. Acad. Sci., 1950, 231, pp. 184-186.

4. - F. GROS, M. BELJANSKI, M. MACHEBOEUF,« Action de la pénicilline sur le métabolisme de l'acide ribonucléique chez Staphylococcus aureus ». Bull. Soc. Chim. Biol., 1951, 33, pp.1696-1717.

5. - F. GROS, M. BELJANSKI, M. MACHEBOEUF, F. GRUMBACH, F. BOYER, « Activité biologique des combinaisons streptomycine-acides gras ». C.R. Acad., Sci., 1951, 232, pp.764-766.

6. - M. BELJANSKI, « Etude de souches bactériennes résistantes à des antibiotiques. Comparaison avec des souches sensibles de mêmes espèces ». Ann. Biol., 1951, 27, pp. 775-780.

7. - M. BELJANSKI, « Etude des souches bactériennes résistantes à des antibiotiques. Comparaison avec des souches sensibles de mêmes espèces ». Thèse de Doctorat ès Sciences d'Etat, Université Paris-la Sorbonne, 1951, Paris, Librairie Arnette, 1952.

8. - M. BELJANSKI, « Action de la cocarboxylase sur le métabolisme des acides nucléiques chez Staphylococcus aureus sensible et résistant à la streptomycine ». 2ème Congrès Intern. de Biochimie, Paris, 1952. Résumé des communications, 99.

9. - M. BELJANSKI, « Comparaison de souches bactériennes résistantes à des antibiotiques avec des souches sensibles de même espèce -I : Cas de la streptomycine ». Ann. Inst. Pasteur, 1952, 83, pp. 80-101.

10. - M. BELJANSKI, « Comparaison de souches bactériennes résistantes à des antibiotiques avec des souches sensibles de même espèce - II : Cas de la pénicilline ». Ann. Inst. Pasteur, 1953, 84, pp. 402-408.

11. - M. BELJANSKI, « Comparaison de souches bactériennes résistantes à des antibiotiques avec des souches sensibles de même espèce -III : Cas du sulfamide - IV : Cas de l'azoture de sodium ». Ann. Inst. Pasteur, 1953, 84, pp. 756-764.

12. - M. BELJANSKI, « Comparaison de souches bactériennes résistantes à la streptomycine avec des souches sensibles de même espèce ». C.R. Acad. Sci., 1953, 236, pp. 1102-1104.

13. - M. BELJANSKI, F. GRUMBACH, « Etude biochimique d'une souche de Mycobacterium tuberculosis streptomycino-sensible et d'une souche streptomycino-résistance dérivée de la souche sensible ». C.R. Acad., Sci., 1953, 236, pp. 2111-2113.

14. - M. BELJANSKI, « Etude des acides nucléiques de souches bactériennes résistantes à la streptomycine et souches de mêmes espèces mais sensibles à l'antibiotique ». Ann. Inst. Pasteur, 1953, 85, pp. 463-469.

15. - M. BELJANSKI, J.GUELFI, « Etude à l'aide du 32P de l'accumulation des acides nucléiques chez Staphylococcus aureus et Salmonella enteritidis résistants et sensibles à la streptomycine ». Ann. Inst. Pasteur, 1954, 86, pp. 115-117.

16. - M. BELJANSKI, « L'absence de cytochromes et de certains systèmes enzymatiques dans un nouveau mutant d'Escherichia coli streptomycino-résistant. Comparaison avec la souche sensible dont il dérive ». C.R. Acad., Sci., 1954, 238, pp. 852-854.

17. - M. BELJANSKI, « L'action de la ribonucléase et de la désoxyribonucléase sur l'incorporation de glycocolle radioactif dans les protéines de lysats de Micrococcus lysodeikticus ». Biochim. Biophys. Acta. 15, 99. 425-431.

18. - M. BELJANSKI, « Isolement de mutants d'Escherichia coli streptomycino-résistants dépourvus d'enzymes respiratoires. Action de l'hémine sur la formation de ces enzymes chez le mutant H-7 ». C.R. Acad., Sci., 1955, 240, pp. 374-376.

19. - M. BELJANSKI, « Formation d'enzymes respiratoires chez un mutant d'Escherichia coli streptomycino-résistant ne manifestant pas d'activité respiratoire ». 3ème Congrès Intern. Biochim., Bruxelles, 1955, p. 98 - Résumés des communications.

20. - R. LATARJET, M. BELJANSKI, « Photorestoration in porphyrin-less mutants of Escherichia coli ». Microbial Genetic Bulletin, E. Witkin, 1955 - Résumés.

21. - M. BELJANSKI, « Reconstitution in vitro de la catalase ». C.R. Acad., Sci., 1955, 241, pp. 1353-1355.

22. - R. LATARJET, M. BELJANSKI, « Photorestauration de bactéries dépourvues de porphyrines ». Ann. Inst. Pasteur, 1956, 90, pp. 127-132.

23. - M. BELJANSKI, M. S. BELJANSKI, « Sur la formation d'enzymes respiratoires chez un mutant d'Escherichia coli streptomycino-résistant et auxotrophe pour l'hémine ». Ann. Inst. Pasteur, 1957, 92, pp. 396-412.

24. - M. BELJANSKI, S. OCHOA, "Protein bio-synthesis by a cell-free bacterial system" Proc. Nat. Acad. Sci. Biochemistry, 1958, 44, pp. 494-500.

25. - M. BELJANSKI, M. S. BELJANSKI, VII-ème Congrès Intern. de Microbiol. Stockholm, 1958, Symposium, II. Discussions.

26. - M. BELJANSKI, S. OCHOA, "Protein bio-synthesis by a cell-free bacterial system" IV-ème Congrès Intern. Biochim. Vienne, 1958, p. 49 - Résumés des communications.

27. - M. BELJANSKI, S. OCHOA, "Protein bio-synthesis by a cell-free bacterial system. II-Further studies on the amino acid incorporation enzyme". Proc. Nat. Acad. Sci., 1958, 44, pp. 1157-1161.

28. - M. BELJANSKI, « Identification de quatre kinases spécifiques des diphosphonucléosides dans une préparation enzymatique d'origine bactérienne ». C.R. Acad. Sci., 1959, 248, pp. 1146-1448.

29. - M. BELJANSKI, « Synthèse de peptides par un système enzymatique en présence de nucléoside - triphosphates ». C.R. Acad. Sci., 1960, 250, pp. 624-626.

30. - M. BELJANSKI, "Protein biosynthesis by a cell-free bacterial system. III- Determination of new peptide bonds; requirements for the 'amino acid incorporation enzyme' in protein biosynthesis" Biochim. Biophys. Acta., 1960, 41, pp. 104-110.

31. - M. BELJANSKI, "Protein biosynthesis by a cell-free bacterial system. IV- Exchange of diphosphonucleosides with homologous triphosphonucleosides by the amino acid incorporation enzyme". Biochim. Biophys. Acta., 1960, 41, pp. 111-115.

32. - M. BELJANSKI, "Ribonucleoside-5'-triphosphate dependent synthesis of peptides by the purified amino acid incorporation enzyme". Progress in Biophysics and Biophysical Chemistry, Pergamon Press, 1961, 11, p. 238.

33. - M. BELJANSKI, « Ribonucléoside-triphosphates et synthèses de peptides spécifiques par des enzymes purifiés ». Bull. Soc. Chim. Biol., 1961,43, pp. 1018-1030.

34. - M. BELJANSKI, « Ribonucléoside-triphosphates et synthèse enzymatique de liaisons peptidiques ». Symposium sur les Acides Ribonucléiques et les Polyphosphates ». C.N.R.S., 1961, pp. 474-475.

35. - M. BELJANSKI, M. S. BELJANSKI, « Synthèses de peptides spécifiques par un système enzymatique purifié d'Alcaligenes faecalis ». Vème Congrès Intern. Biochim. Moscou, 1961, p. 24.

36. - M. BELJANSKI, Discussions, Symposium sur la Biosynthèse des Protéines. Vème Congrès Intern. Biochim. Moscou, 1961.

37. - J.P. ZALTA, M. BELJANSKI, « Synthèse de peptides par des fractions subcellulaires préparées à partir du foie de rat ». C.R. Acad. Sci. 1961, 253, pp. 567-569

38. - M. BELJANSKI, M. S. BELJANSKI, T. LOVINY, « Rôle des polypeptide-synthétases dans la formation de peptides spécifiques en présence de ribonucléoside-triphosphates ». Biochim. Biophys. Acta., 1962, 56, pp. 559-570.

39. - M. BELJANSKI, « Participation of an RNA fraction in peptide synthesis in the presence of a purified enzyme system from Alcaligenes faecalis ». Biochim. Biophys. Res. Comm., 1962, 8, pp. 15-19.

40. - M. BELJANSKI, M. S. BELJANSKI, « Acide aminé - acide ribonucléique , intermédiaire dans la synthèse des liasons peptidiques ». VI- Biochim. Biophys. Acta., 1963, 72, pp. 585-597.

41. - M. BELJANSKI, « ARN-messager: intermédiaire direct dans la synthèse des liaisons peptidiques ». Colloque International du C.N.R.S., Marseille, 1963, pp. 39-44. (Mécanismes de régulation des activités cellulaires chez les micro-organismes).

42. - M. BELJANSKI, C. FISHER, M. S. BELJANSKI, « Le RNA messager, accepteur spécifique des L-acides aminés en présence d'enzymes bactériennes ». C.R. Acad. Sci., 1963,257, pp. 547-549.

43. - M. BELJANSKI, C. FISHER, « Les ARN messagers gouvernant la synthèse « in vitro » des chaînes peptidiques en présence de polypeptides synthétases ». Pathologie-Biologie, 1965,13, pp. 198-203.

44. - M. BELJANSKI, "Messenger RNA dependent Synthesis of peptides by purified bacterial enzymes". Bioch-Zeits, 1965, 342, pp. 392-399.

45. - M. BELJANSKI, « L'ARN isolé du virus de la mosaïque jaune du Navet, accepteur des l-acides aminés en présence d'enzymes bactériennes ». Bull. Soc. Chim. Biol. 1965, 47, pp. 1645-1652.

46. - M. BELJANSKI, N. VAPAILLE, « Rôle des triterpènes dans l'attachement des l-acides aminés par des « ARN matriciels » ». Eur. J. of Clin. Biol. Res., 1971, pp. 897-908.

47. - M. BELJANSKI, P. BOURGAREL, « Isolement de di- et trinucléotides, sites spécifiques d'attachement d'arginine et de valine dans des ARN d' origines différentes ». C.R. Acad. Sci., 1967, 264, pp. 1760-1763 (série D).

48. - M. BELJANSKI, C. FISCHER-FERRARO, « Nouvelle méthode de purification des polypeptides synthétases ». C.R. Acad. Sci., 1967, 264, pp. 411-414 (série D).

49. - M. BELJANSKI, C. FISCHER-FERRARO, P. BOURGAREL, « Identification des sites d'attachement spécifiques d'arginine et de valine dans des ARN d' origines différentes ». VIII- European J. Biochem., 1968, 4, pp. 184-189.

50. - C. FISCHER-FERRARO, M. BELJANSKI, « Nouvelle méthode de purification des polypeptides synthétases ». VII- European J. Biochem., 1968, 4, pp. 118-125.

51. - M. BELJANSKI, P. BOURGAREL, « Isolement et caractérisation d'un RNA matriciel d'Alcaligenes faecalis ». C.R. Acad. Sci., 1968, 266, pp. 845-847.

52. - M. BELJANSKI, M.S. BELJANSKI, « Synthèse chez Escherichia coli des ARN dont la structure primaire diffère de celle de l'ADN ». C.R. Acad. Sci., 1968, 267, pp. 1058-1060 (série D).

53. - M. BELJANSKI, M.S. BELJANSKI, P. BOURGAREL, J. CHASSAGNE, « Synthèse chez les bactéries d'ARN nouveaux n'étant pas la copie de l'ADN ». C.R. Acad. Sci., 1969, 269, pp. 240-243 (série D).

54. - M. BELJANSKI, P. BOURGAREL, M.S. BELJANSKI, « Showdomycine et biosynthèse d'ARN non complémentaire de l'ADN » - I -. Ann. Inst. Pasteur, 1970, 118, pp. 253-276.

55. - M. BELJANSKI, P. BOURGAREL, M.S. BELJANSKI, "Drastic alteration of ribosomal RNA and ribosomal proteins in showdomycin-resistant Escherichia Coli". Proc. Nat. Aca. Sci. (USA), 1971,68, pp. 491-495.

56. - M. PLAWECKI, M. BELJANSKI, « Transcription par la polynucléotide phosphorylase de l'ARN associé à l'ADN d'Escherichia coli ». C.R. Acad. Sci., 1971, 273, pp. 827-830 (série D).

57. - M. BELJANSKI, M.S. BELJANSKI, P. BOURGAREL, « ARN transformants porteurs de caractères héréditaires chez Escherichia coli showdomycino-résistant ». C.R. Acad. Sci., 1971, 272, pp. 2107-2110 (série D).

58. - M. BELJANSKI, M.S. BELJANSKI, P. BOURGAREL, « « Episome à ARN » porté par l'ADN d'Escherichia coli sauvage et showdomycino-résistant ». C.R. Acad. Sci., 1971, 272, pp. 2736-3739 (série D).

59. - M. BELJANSKI, M.S. BELJANSKI, P. MANIGAULT, P. BOURGAREL, "Transformation of Agrobacterium tumefaciens into a non-oncogenic species by an Escheria coli RNA" Proc. Nat. Aca. Sci. (USA), 1972, 69, pp. 191-195.

60. - M. BELJANSKI, « Synthèse in vitro de l'ADN sur une matrice d'ARN par une transcriptase d'Escherichia coli ». C.R. Acad. Sci., 1972, 274, pp.2801-2804 (série D).

61. - M. BELJANSKI, C. BONISSOL, P. KONA, « Transformation des cellules K.B. induites par la showdomycine ». C.R. Acad. Sci., 1972,274, pp. 3116-3119 (série D).

62. - M. BELJANSKI, P. MANIGAULT, "Genetic transformation of bacteria by RNA and loss of oncogenic power properties of Agrobacterium tumefaciens. Transforming RNA as template for DNA synthesis". Sixth Miles International Symposium on Molecular Biology. Ed. F. Beers and R.C. Tilghman. The John Hopkins University Press, Baltimore, 1972, pp. 81-97.

63. - M. BELJANSKI, « Séparation de la transcriptase inverse de l'ADN polymérase ADN dépendante. Analyse de l'ADN synthétisé sur le modèle de l'ARN transformant ». C.R. Acad. Sci., 1973, 276, pp. 1625-1628 (série D).

64. - M. BELJANSKI, M. PLAWECKI, "Transforming RNA as a template directing RNA and DNA synthesis in bacteria". In Niu and Segal (eds), The Role of RNA in Reproduction and Development. North Holland Publ.Co., 1973, pp. 203-224.

65. - M. PLAWECKI, M. BELJANSKI, « Synthèse in vitro d'un ARN utilisé comme amorceur pour la réplication de l'ADN ». C.R. Acad. Sci., 1974, 278, pp. 1413-1416 (série D).

66. - M. BELJANSKI, Y. AARON-DA-CUNHA, M.S. BELJANSKI, P. MANIGAULT, P. BOURGAREL, "Isolation of the tumor-inducing RNA

from Oncogenic and Nononcogenic Agrobacterium tumefaciens". Proc. Nat. Acad. Sci. (USA), 1974,71, pp. 1585-1589.

67. - M. BELJANSKI, M.S. BELJANSKI, « RNA-bound Reverse Transcriptase in Escherichia coli and *in vitro* synthesis of a complementary DNA ». Biochemical genetics, 1974, 12, pp. 163-180.

68. - M. BELJANSKI, P. MANIGAULT, M.S. BELJANSKI, Y. AARON-DA-CUNHA, "Genetic transformation of Agrobacterium tumefaciens by RNA and nature of the tumor inducing principle". First Intern. Congress of the Intern. Assoc. of Microbiol. Soc. Tokyo I.A.M.S., 1974,1, pp.132-141.

69. - M. BELJANSKI, M. S. BELJANSKI, M. PLAWECKI, P. MANI-GAULT, « ARN-fragments, amorceurs nécessaires à la réplication « in vitro » des ADN ». C.R. Acad. Sci., 1975,280, pp. 363-366 (série D).

70. - M. BELJANSKI, L. CHAUMONT, C. BONISSOL, M. S. BELJANSKI, « ARN-fragments inhibiteurs « in vivo » de la multiplication des virus du fibrome de Shope et de la vaccine » C.R. Acad. Sci., 1975, 280, pp. 783-786 (série D).

71. - M. BELJANSKI, « ARN-amorceurs riches en nucléotides G et A indispensables à la réplication *in vitro* de l'ADN des phages YX174 et lambda ». C.R. Acad. Sci., 1975, 280, pp. 783-786 (série D).

72. - L. LE GOFF, Y. AARON-DA-CUNHA, M. BELJANSKI, "RNA fraction from several nononcogenic strains of Agrobacterium tumefaciens as tumor inducing agent in Datura stramonium". XIIth Intern. Bot. Congress. Résumés. Leningrad, 1975.

73. - M. BELJANSKI, Y. AARON-DA-CUNHA, "RNA fraction from others sources than Agrobacterium tumefaciens as tumor inducing agent in Datura stramonium". Workshop Third Intern. Congress of Virology, Madrid, 1975, p. 15.

74 . - L. LE GOFF, Y. AARON-DA-CUNHA, M. BELJANSKI, « Un ARN extrait d'Agrobacterium tumefaciens souches oncogènes et non oncogènes, éléments indispensables à l'induction des tumeurs chez Datura stramonium ». Canadian J. of Microbiology, 1976, 22, pp. 694-701.

75. - M. BELJANSKI, Y. AARON-DA-CUNHA, "Particular small size RNA and RNA fragments from different origins as tumor inducing agents in in Datura stramoium". Molec. Biol. Reports, 1976, 2, pp. 497-506.

76. S.K. DUTTA, M. BELJANSKI, P. BOURGAREL, "Endogenous RNA-bound RNA dependent DNA polymerase activity in Neurospora crassa". Exp. Mycology, 1977, 1, pp. 173-182.

77. L. LE GOFF, Y. AARON-DA-CUNHA, M. BELJANSKI, « Polyribonucleotides, agents inducteurs et inhibiteurs des tissus tumoraux ». Conf. Intern. Montpellier (1978) - Résumés.

78. - M. BELJANSKI, P. BOURGAREL, M.S. BELJANSKI, « Découpage des ARN ribosomiques d'Escherichia coli par la ribonucléase U2 et transcription *in vitro* des ARN-fragments en ADN complémentaires ». C.R. Acad. Sci., 1978, 286, pp. 1825-1828 (série D).

79. - M. BELJANSKI, M. PLAWECKI, P. BOURGAREL, M. S. BELJANSKI, « Nouvelles substances (R.L.B.) actives dans la leucopoïese et la formation des plaquettes ». Bull. Acad. Nat. Med., 1978, 162, Volume n°6, pp. 475-781.

80. - M. STROUN, Ph. ANKER, M. BELJANSKI, J. HENRI, Ch. LEDERREY, M. OJHA, P. MAURICE, "Presence of RNA in the nucleo-protein complex spontaneously released by human lymphocytes and frog auricles". Cancer Res., 1978, 38, pp. 3546-3551.

81. - M. BELJANSKI, L. LE GOFF, Y. AARON-DA-CUNHA, "Special short dual-action RNA fragments can both induce and inhibit

crown-gall tumors". Proc. 4th Conf. Plant Path. Bacteria Angers, 1978, pp. 207-220.

82. - M. BELJANSKI, L. LE GOFF, « Stimulation de l'induction - ou inhibition du développement - des tumeurs de crown-gall par des ARN-fragments U2. Interférence de l'auxine ». C.R. Acad. Sci., 1979, 288, pp. 147-150 (série D).

83. - M. BELJANSKI, M. PLAWECKI, "Particular RNA fragments as promoters of leucocytes and platelet formations in rabbits". Exp. Cell Biol., 1979, 47, pp. 218-225.

84. - M. BELJANSKI, "Oncotest: a DNA assay system for the screening of carcinogenic substances". IRCS Medical science, 1979, 47, pp. 218-225.

85. - L. LE GOFF, M. BELJANSKI, "Cancer/anti-cancer dual action drugs in crown-gall tumors". IRCS Medical Science, 1979,7, p. 476.

86. - M. BELJANSKI, "Oligoribo-nucleotides, promoters of leucocyte and platelet genesis in animals depleted by anticancer drugs". NCI-EORTC Symposium on nature, prevention and treatment of clinical toxicity of anticancer agents. Institut Bordet, Bruxelles, 1980.

87. - M. BELJANSKI, M. PLAWECKI, P. BOURGAREL, M.S. BELJANSKI, "Short chain RNA fragments as promoters of leucocyte and platelet genesis in animals depleted by anti-cancer drugs". In the Role of RNA in Development and Reproduction. Sec. Int. Symposium, April 25-30, 1980, pp. 79-113. Science Press Beijing. M.C. Niu and H.H. Chuang Eds Van Nostrand Reinhold Company.

88. - M. BELJANSKI, P. BOURGAREL, M.S. BELJANSKI, "Correlation between *in vitro* DNA synthesis, DNA strand separation and in vivo multiplication of cancer cells". Expl. Cell. Biol., 49,1981, pp.220-231.

89. - M. PLAWECKI, M. BELJANSKI, "Comparative study of Escherichia coli endotoxin, hydrocortisone and Beljanski Leucocyte

Restorers activity in cyclophosphamide-treated rabbits". Proc. of the Soc. for Exp. Biol. and Med., 168, 1981, pp.408-413.

90. - M. BELJANSKI, L. LE GOFF, M.S. BELJANSKI, "Differential susceptibility of cancer and normal DNA templates allows the detection of carcinogens and anticancer drugs". Third NCI-EORTS Symp. on new drugs in Cancer Therapy, Institut Bordet, Bruxelles, 1981.

91. - L. LE GOFF, M. BELJANSKI, "Crown-gall tumor stimulation or inhibition: correlation with DNA strand separation". Proc. Fifth Conf. Plant Path. Bact. Cali, 1981, p. 295-307.

92. - M. BELJANSKI, M.S. BELJANSKI, "Selective inhibition of *in vitro* synthesis of cancer DNA by alkaloids of b-carboline class". Expl. Cell. Biol., 50, 1982, pp.79-87.

93. - L. LE GOFF, M. BELJANSKI, « Agonist and/or antagonists effects of plant hormones and an anticancer alkaloid on plant structure and activity » IRCS Med. Sci., 10, 1982, pp. 689-690.

94. - M. BELJANSKI, L. LE GOFF, A. FAIVRE-AMIOT, « Preventive and curative anticancer drug. Application to Crown-gall tumors » Acta Horticulturae, n°125, 1982, pp. 239-248.

95. - M. BELJANSKI, « Oncotest: dépistage des potentiels cancérogènes et spécifiquement cancéreux. Conceptions et perspectives nouvelles en cancérologie ». Environnement et nouvelle médecine. n°2, 1982, pp.18-23.

96. - M. BELJANSKI, L. LE GOFF, M. S. BELJANSKI, « In vitro Screening of Carcinogens using DNA of the His-Mutant of Salmonella typhimurium ». Expl. Cell. Biol., 50, 1982, pp. 271-280.

97. - M. BELJANSKI, L. LE GOFF, « Tumor promoter (TPA), DNA chain opening and unscheduled DNA synthesis ». IRCS Med. Sci., 11, 1983, pp. 363-364.

98. - M. BELJANSKI, M. PLAWECKI, P. BOURGAREL, M.S. BELJANSKI, « Leucocyte recovery whith short-chain RNA fragments in cyclophosphamide-treated rabbits ». Cancer Treatment Reports, 67, 1983, pp. 611-619.

99. - M. BELJANSKI, « The Regulation of DNA Replication and Transcription. The Role of Trigger Molecules in Normal and Malignant Gene Expression ». Experimental Biology and Medicine, vol. 8, Karger (1983), pp. 1-190.

100. - M. BELJANSKI, M.S. BELJANSKI, « Three alkaloids as selective destroyers of the proliferative capacity of cancer cells ». IRCS Med. Sci., 12, 1984, pp. 587-588.

101. - L. LE GOFF, J. ROUSSAUX, Y. AARON-DA-CUNHA, M. BELJANSKI, « Growth inhibition of crown-gall tissues in relation to the structure and activity of DNA » Physiol. Plant., 64, 1985, pp 177-184.

102. - L. LE GOFF, M. BELJANSKI, « The *in vitro* effects of opines and other compounds on DNAs originating from bacteria and from healthy and tumorous plant tissues ». Expl. Cell. Biol., 53, 1985, pp. 335-350.

103. - M. BELJANSKI, « Activation et inactivation des gènes: Incidence en cancérologie ». Aspect de la recherche. Université Paris-Sud, 1985, pp. 56-62.

104. - M. BELJANSKI, M.S. BELJANSKI, « Three alkaloids as selective destroyers of cancer cells in mice. Synergy with classic anticancer drugs ». Oncology, 43, 1986, pp 198-203.

105. - M. BELJANSKI, L. LE GOFF, « Analysis of small RNA species: phylogenetic trends ». In DNA Systematics, vol.I: Evolution. Ed. S.K. Dutta CRC Press, Inc. Florida (1986), pp.81-105.

106. - M. BELJANSKI, T. NAWROCKI, L. LE GOFF, « Possible role of markers synthesized during cancer evolution: I- Markers in mammalien tissues ». IRCS Med. Sci. 14, 1986, pp. 809-810.

107. - L. LE GOFF, M. BELJANSKI, « Possible role of markers synthesized during cancer evolution: II- Markers in crown-gall tissues ». IRCS Med. Sci. 14, 1986, pp. 811-812.

108. - M. BELJANSKI, L. LE GOFF, M.S. BELJANSKI, « Régulation des gènes, cancer et prévention ». Médecines nouvelles, 15, 1986, pp. 57-86.

109. - M. BELJANSKI, « Terminal deoxynucleotidyl transferase and ribonuclease activities in purified hepatitis-B antigen ». Med. Sci. Res., 15, 1987, pp. 529-530.

110. - M. BELJANSKI, S.K. DUTTA, « Differential synthesis and replication of DNA in the Neurospora crassa slime mutant versus normal cells: Role of carcinogens ». Oncology, 44, 1987, pp. 327-330.

111. - S.K. DUTTA, M. BELJANSKI, « Particular RNA primer from growth medium differentially stimulates *in vitro* DNA synthesis and in vivo cell growth of Neurospora crassa and its slime mutant ». Current Genetics, 12, 1987, pp. 283-289.

112. - M. BELJANSKI, L.C. NIU, M.S. BELJANSKI, S. YAN, M.C. NIU, « Iron stimulated RNA-dependent DNA polymerase Activity from goldfish eggs ». Cellular and Molecular Biology, 34, 1988, pp. 17-25.

113. - L. LE GOFF, M. WICKER, M. BELJANSKI, « Reversible biophysical changes of DNAs from *in vitro* culturel non-tumour cells ». Med. Sci. Res., 16, 1988, pp. 359-360.

114. - M. STROUN, P. ANKER, P. MAURICE, J. LYAUTEY, C. LEDER-REY, M. BELJANSKI, « Neoplastic Characteristics of the DNA Found in the Plasma of Cancer Patients ». Oncology, 16, 1989, pp. 318-322.

115. - M. BELJANSKI, M.S. BELJANSKI, M. GRANDI « Resultati preliminari dell'impiego di tre alcaloidi nel carcinoma prostatico ». In Tumori, Instituo Nationale per le studio ed la cura dei tumori (ed. Lambrosiana), Vol. 75, suppl. 4, 1989.

116. - M. BELJANSKI, « Cancer therapy: A New Approach ». Deutsche Zeitschrift für Onkologie 5, 22, 1990, pp. 145-152.

117. - M. BELJANSKI, « Cancer et Sida. Nouvelles approches thérapeutiques ». 5èmes Entretiens Internationaux de Monaco, 21-24 novembre 1990 (Ed. du Rocher), pp. 25-34.

118. - D. DONADIO, R. LORHO, J.E. CAUSSE, T. NAWROCKI, M. BELJANSKI, « RNA fragments (RLB) and Tolerance of Cytostatic Treatments in Hematology: A Preliminary Study about Two Non-Hodgkin Malignant Lymphoma Cases ». Deutsche Zeitschrift für Onkologie, 23, 2, 1991, pp. 33-35.

119. - M. BELJANSKI, « Reverse Transcriptases in Bacteria: Small RNAs as Genetic Vectors and Biological Modulators ». Brazil. J. Genetics, 14, 4, 1991, pp. 873-896.

120. - M. BELJANSKI, « Radioprotection of Irradiated Mice - Mechanisms and Synergistic Action of WR-2721 and R.L.B. ». Deutsche Zeitschrift für Onkologie, 23, 6, 1991, pp. 155-159.

121. - M. BELJANSKI, « Overview: BLRs as Inducers of in vivo Leucocyte and Platelet Genesis ». Deutsche Zeitschrift für Onkologie, 24, 2, 1992, pp. 45-45.

122. - M. BELJANSKI, « A New Approach to Cancer Therapy ». Proceedings of the international seminar: Traditional Medicine: A Challenge of the 21st Century, 7-9 Nov. 1992, Calcutta (Ed. in chief Biswapati Mukherjee).

123. - M. BELJANSKI, S. CROCHET, M.S. BELJANSKI, « PB100: A Potent and Selective Inhibitor of Human BCNU Resistant Glioblastoma Cell Multiplication ». Anticancer Research, vol. 13, n°6A, Nov. Dec. 1993, pp. 2301-2308.

124. - M. BELJANSKI, S. CROCHET, « Differential effects of ferritin, calcium, zinc and gallic acid on *in vitro* proliferation of human

glioblastoma cells and normal astrocytes ». J. Lab. Clin. Med. 123:547-555, 1994.

125. - M. BELJANSKI, S. CROCHET, « The selective anticancer agent PB-100 inhibits interleukin-6 induced enhancement of glioblastoma cell proliferation in vitro ». International Journal of Oncology, 5:873-879, 1994.

126. - M. BELJANSKI, S. CROCHET, « Selective inhibitor (PB-100) of human glioblastoma cell multiplication ». Journal of Neuro-Oncology, Vol. 21, N°1, p. 62, 1994.

127. - J.E. CAUSSE, T. NAWROCKI, M. BELJANSKI, « Human Skin Fibrosis Rnase Search for a Biological Inhibitor-Regulator ». Deutsche Zeitschrift für Onkologie, 26, 5, 1994, pp. 137-139.

128. - M. BELJANSKI, S. CROCHET, « The anticancer agent PB100 concentrates in the nucleus and nucleoli of human glioblastoma cells but does not enter normal astrocytes ». International Journal of Oncology 7:81-85, 1995.

129. - M. BELJANSKI, « Novel selective non-toxic anticancer and antiviral agents ». International Journal of Oncology Vol. 7. supplement, p. 983, October 1995.

130. - M. BELJANSKI, S. CROCHET, « The selective anticancer agents PB-100 and BG-8 are active against human melanoma cells, but do not affect non malignant fibroblasts ». International Journal of Oncology 8:1143-1148, 1996.

131. - M. BELJANSKI, S. CROCHET, « Mitogenic effect of several interleukins, neuromediators and hormones on human glioblastoma cells, and its inhibition by the selective anticancer agent PB-100 ». Deutsche Zeitschrift für Onkologie, 28, 1, 1996, pp. 14-2.

132. - M. BELJANSKI, « De novo synthesis of DNA - like molecules by polyaudeotide phosphorylase in vitro ». J. Mol. Evol. 1996, 42:493-499.

133. - M. BELJANSKI, « The anticancer agent PB-100, selectively active on malignant cells, inhibits multiplication of sixteen malignant cell lines, even multidrug resistant. » Genetics and Molecular Biology, 23, 1, 29-33 (2000).

About the Author

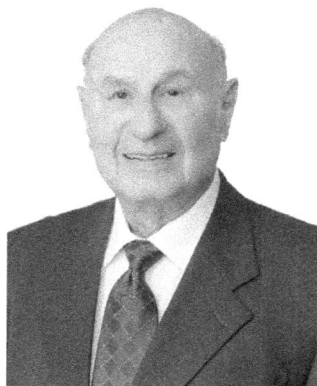

Dr. Morton Walker, D.P.M., is a professional medical journalist who has authored 92 published books, 14 of which are bestsellers, and over 2000 clinical journal and magazine articles about holistic medicine, orthomolecular nutrition, and other alternative methods of healing. Named "The World's Leading Medical Journalist Specializing In Holistic Medicine" by the American Cancer Control Society, Dr. Walker lives and conducts his medical journalism research in Florida. He is the recipient of 23 medical journalism awards for his breakthrough works in many areas including longevity, chelation therapies, and cancer. Dr. Walker's most recent works, including *The Gerson Therepies* coauthored with Charlotte Gerson, *The Yeast Syndrome: How to Help Your Doctor Identify & Treat the Real Cause of Your Yeast-Related Illness* coauthored with John P. Trowbridge, and *Olive Leaf Extract*, have all sold over one million copies.

For more information on Dr. Morton Walker and his work, please visit *www.DrMortonWalker.com*.